PUBLISHER

Published in the UK by Medicause
Medical Information & Medical Science Publisher,
115 High Rd., Loughton, Essex IG10 4JA UK

www.daviddighton.com
email: david@daviddighton.com

DEDICATION

This book is dedicated
to my son Nicholas, and to my daughters
Anna and Florence
and all my former
patients, teachers and colleagues.

ABOUT THE AUTHOR

Dr. David H. Dighton qualified at the London Hospital Medical College in 1966 with MB and BS (London) degrees. In 1970, after a short time in NHS general practice, he became a British Heart Foundation Fellow in Cardiology at St. George's Hospital Hyde Park Corner, London, working with cardiologists Dr Aubrey Leatham and Dr Alan Harris. In 1973, he became a MRCP(UK), and later became a Lecturer (London University) in Medicine and Cardiology at Charing Cross Hospital, London.

In 1980, the Vrije University Hospital in Amsterdam appointed him as Chef de Clinique (Assistant Professor). Having returned to the UK in1982, he worked both in his own private medical practice in Loughton, Essex (The Loughton Clinic, was initially established in 1973 as a medical nursing home), and at the Wellington Hospital, London. In 2000, he started a private diagnostic cardiac centre specialising in heart disease prevention and the early detection of heart and artery disease (The Cardiac Centre Loughton).

He retired from practice aged 76-years, having been a medical student and doctor for 58 years. His retirement followed many conflicts with three medical regulators. He had disagreements with them about how medicine should be practised, and who is most qualified to regulate and supervise it. Observing the progressive demise of the NHS in the UK, he remains in disagreement with them; views expressed in his book, *The NHS. Our Sick Sacred Cow.* 2023.

DOCTORS, NURSES AND PATIENTS

HOW TO SURVIVE MEDICAL PRACTICE

DR DAVID H. DIGHTON

BOOKS BY THE SAME AUTHOR

*Eat to Your Heart's Content. The diet and lifestyle for a healthy heart.***(2003).** HeartShield.
  ISBN: 0-9551072-0-2

*HeartSense.How to look after your heart.***(2006). HeartShield.**
  ISBN: 0-9551072-1-0

The NHS: Our Sick Sacred Cow: Causes and Cures (2023)
  ISBN: 978-1-3999-6027-4 (also ebook).

How to Become Heart-Smart. A User's Guide to Hear Health and Heart Disease Prevention. (2023 1st Ed./2nd Ed. 2024. ISBN: 978-1-3999-7461-5 (also ebook).

Who Loses Wins. Winning Weight Loss Battles: A 'Fat Mentality' v A 'Fit Mentality' **(2024).**
  ISBN: 978-1-7385207-1-8 (ebook: 978-1-7385207-2-5)

In Preparation: *The Art and Science of Medicine and Essential Cardiology for Students.*

CONTACT

For more information, go to 'www.daviddighton.com' or email: david@daviddighton.com or daviddighton@loughtonclinic.org

CONTENTS

Introduction

Doctors, nurses and patients need to understand one another. With that in mind, this book describes the many characters each can portray.

When considered as characters, doctors and nurses each play their role in different ways, and will manage medical conditions in ways that not only affect a patient's quality of life but also their morbidity and mortality.

Doctors and nurses gain an advantage when they understand their patients well, and patients benefit from understanding what difference various types of doctor and nurse can make to their life.

Doctors and nurses are not all equally effective in treating people, and patients deserve to know why. This book aims to enable doctors to better understand those they treat and help patients to decide who should treat them.

Some doctors and nurses prefer to treat patients as numbers, but most want to treat patients as sentient human beings. Many specialist doctors now only treat specific problems, whereas once we had general physicians and surgeons capable of much more. GPs alone have kept their ability to treat all-comers.

Although I have focussed on doctors and nurses, I must acknowledge that many others care for patients. They include pharmacists, hairdressers, carers, counsellors, social workers, paramedics and friends. They can assume that my descriptions represent them.

Over the five decades I practised as a general physician and cardiologist, I met many doctors, nurses and thousands of patients, each with their own needs, and their own particular attitude and outlook.

I first became fascinated by how doctors worked while watching early TV programmes. Emergency Ward 10 was the first that interested me. Later came *Dr Finlay's Casebook*, and *Dr Kildare*. The patients, doctors and nurses were then all Caucasian with no mention of race and culture. Although these need to be discussed, the doctor-patient relationship remains the founding bedrock of good medical practice. Within, I describe its important aspects.

In the days before coloured TV, patients had relationships with doctors that were more formal than today. Doctors then came from rich educated families, and many had experienced the work of their mother or father as a doctor. Medicine was a middle-class vocation. Those who became nurses and doctors then represented those given to public duty, and not to business. Their aim was to serve. Many would have pursued their vocation, even if unpaid.

Doctors, nurses and patients today are now drawn from different classes and cultures, and understanding one another has become an issue. Since diagnoses come mostly from the history patients provide, problems with understanding (language and culture), are a challenge for all involved.

As far as I can tell, patients did not change over the fifty-three years I practised as a doctor, although they are now much more aware of dangers: tired doctors, insufficient services available at weekends, difficult to get GP appointments, and NHS emergency services stretched to the limit.

Medical bureaucrats now tacitly suggest that every doctor is a potential Dr. Harold Shipman, and every nurse a potential Lucy Letby, until proven otherwise. The result has been that doctors and nurses have changed their approach to patients. Some now see all patients as potential litigants. Everything doctors and nurses do now has a medico-legal dimension. Everything said and done, needs to be recorded and audited for the satisfaction of managers with MBAs and law degrees, many of whom are better qualified to run business corporations than NHS medical facilities. As a result, the focus of some nurses and doctors has had to move away from patient care to corporate management compliance.

Bureaucracy has raised patient expectations in the UK, while the services provided have steadily become less accessible.

The conditions under which doctors and nurses work is important to the quality of care they can give, so some mention of them is obligatory. The NHS is dysfunctional in many parts of Britain, with doctors and nurses being portrayed as responsible when they are not. The blame lies with government officials and the thousands of bureaucrats who organise medical practice, many with no knowledge or understanding of medical or surgical practice. Who, I wonder, gave them power over nurses and doctors? And who would want their Army run by lawyers, accountants and business people rather than experienced soldiers? The equivalent in UK medical practice, doctors, nurses and patients now have to put up with. Both represent an insult to stupidity, and it is no surprise that many doctors and nurses now seek to emigrate (Drexit).

My hope is for each doctor, patient and nurse to better understand one another. I hope the information given is both useful and amusing.

CHAPTER ONE

DOCTORS AND NURSES AS CHARACTERS

Nothing can replace a good heart and a sensible head.

Yehudi Menuhin

There are some important questions to consider about the character of doctors. Are there many types of doctor? What character have they, and of what significance is their character to patient welfare and their professional relationships?

What follows is incomplete. It would be impossible to describe every type of doctor, although I have drawn on fifty-three years of experiencing them to write this. Most doctors are affable and good at their job; these I have described only briefly. There are, however, many exceptions.

It is these exceptions I have focussed on as a forewarning to patients.

I have tried to follow in the footsteps of Theophrastus, an associate of Aristotle, who described the various Greek characters he met 2300 years ago. I cannot emulate Shakespeare, who brought every variation of human nature before us in his plays, or Dickens, who populated his novels with every conceivable character. Every canon of literature is replete with many more character descriptions.

I have created some acronyms that are meant to amuse and serve as a diplomatic device for doctors communicating with one another.

Types of Nurses and Doctors

Dr. Kate Granger, who died in 2016, was astounded to find that when she was ill herself, some hospital doctors failed to introduce themselves as they approached her hospital bed. She started a campaign: '#HelloMyNameIs'. She hoped NHS doctors would consider patients as people, and not just disease entities.

Theophrastus, in the 3rd century BC, wrote his 'Characters', eloquently describing the behaviour of thirty different human types: the dissembler, flatterer, coward, over-zealous, tactless, shameless, newsmonger, mean, stupid, surly, superstitious, thankless, suspicious, disagreeable, exquisite, garrulous, bore, rough, affable, impudent, gross, boorish, penurious, pompous, braggart, oligarch, backbiter, avaricious, the late learner, and the vicious. These types are all still to be found among patients, nurses, and doctors alike. Since human nature has hardly changed, these old truths remain valid.

Of particular importance to every doctor and nurse is to recognise the character of their colleagues: those who are helpful, mean, generous, romantic, practical, and down-to-earth. There are also those with their head in the clouds, and those who see themselves as God's gift to medicine and to procreation. Some are nerds, and some are the life and soul of every party. Some want to be the centre of attention, others are selfish, and self-possessed. It is important to recognise would-be friends, and likely enemies, the knowledgeable, the talented, and those capable of wise counsel. Doctors and nurses will meet them all as colleagues or as patients.

Like St. Paul and St. Thomas Aquinas, those in possession of divine gifts will progress easily. Wisdom, understanding, knowledge, and good counsel are four of St. Paul's seven charismata pertinent to medical professionals.

St. Paul. New Testament Epistles. Corinthians. *The Summa Theologiæ of St. Thomas Aquinas (1225-1274).*

To master a profession, like medicine, requires talent. According to the actor Matt Damon, the film directors Ridley Scott and Clint Eastwood both have features of mastery which could apply to doctors or nurses. He said they had talent, virtuosity, passion and experience. There are doctors and nurses with all these attributes and those with none.

'Every way of a man is right in his own eyes.'
Proverbs 21.2

From a patient's point of view, whether their doctor or nurse is an 'attached' or 'detached' type, carries implications for their welfare. The detached types usually prefer the science of medicine to the art of medicine, but not all know best how to apply them. They will leave the ancient art of medicine to doctors able to feel attached to patients and their problems. The art of medicine defeats regulation and is therefore being side-lined in favour of medical practices which are evidence-based. This is not in every patient's interest, but it is where medical practice is now heading.

The Characters

ABCD

Above and **B**eyond the **C**all of **D**uty. No personal considerations, trivial social arrangements, matters of self-interest, or convenience will divert these dedicated, selfless medical professionals from their work.

In March 2018, the UK experienced Siberian blizzard weather ('Beast from the East'). At this time, Nurse Reg Barker walked ten miles through the snow. He trudged from Crediton to his ward at the Royal Devon and Exeter Hospital to get to work. Reg's action was an example of an ABCD in action.

The Telegraph. 2/3/2018

Abrasives

The typical abrasive doctor asks curt questions and accepts only brief answers. They do not want to waste their time on inconsequential matters. They are usually self-absorbed, time-obsessed, or pressured for time. If they ask, 'Have you noticed any chest tightness on exertion?', they will expect a 'Yes' or 'No' answer, not a narrative description. They do not tolerate garrulousness and will cut patients short. They can be arrogant and forceful, irritable and easily irritated, and can give the impression that they would sooner be somewhere else (and possibly, they should). Perhaps they have missed out on the genes determining generosity, charm, empathy, and sympathy.

Doctors and nurses must prepare well when dealing with them. They must be sure of their facts and argue their case with summarised data. Succinct quotes from research papers will help. They should aim for a knock-out punch.

Do not negotiate out of fear and do not fear to negotiate.
John. F. Kennedy.

In the 17th century, apothecary Nicholas Culpepper, took the patient's point of view, and came into conflict with the physicians of the Royal College (one of whom was William Harvey). Culpepper said, 'no man deserved to starve to pay a proud, insulting, domineering physician'.

Actors

There are many doctors who never became a professional film or stage actor. Instead, some found their way onto hospital wards and into GP surgeries.

Their aim is to create an impression, good enough to enhance their career. As a medical student, one of my surgical consultant tutors was then the ageing Mr. Herman Taylor (he invented a gastroscope). He wore a monocle, and so did his much younger senior registrar (later to become a consultant anaesthetist). The monocle was then useful for non-verbal communication. Allowing it to drop, accompanied by an elevation of the chin and eyebrows, signalled surprise, error and even astonishment. In response to a student answering a question incorrectly, Mr. H.T. could, without saying a word, let all those present know that an error had been made. The amusing thing was that his young senior registrar would attempt the same act in unison (successfully playing the role of young fogey).

Other actors I have known would wear a kilt, or some other apparel, just to grab some limelight. I never actually saw a doctor wearing laurel leaves and a toga, but I suspect there have been those who gave it thought.

Altruists

Many doctors are altruists. Their dedication and self-sacrifice to medicine and research is truly admirable. We need more of them.

The Arrogant

'No good work was ever done by humble men.'

G. H. Hardy, in *A Mathematician's Apology*. (1940).

Arrogance is a common trait among those who pursue power over others. Arrogant medical decision making can be dangerous. Because one can see it in schoolchildren, arrogance is likely to be inherited. The trait is attractive to those biased by an imaginary halos. They may like to bask in the shadow of an alpha, dominant person; one who knows his/her own mind; one who is totally 'in charge', with no doubt about their wisdom or their actions. Arrogance can make the insecure feel secure, even though the basis of their arrogance can itself be insecurity. When the arrogant reject sound advice, merely to justify their status, it can prove fatal.

Arrogance, insolence, and pride are nothing new. Aeschylus wrote about insolence, the arrogance of power and catastrophe:

> 'You see how insolence,
> Once opened into flower,
> Produces fields ripe with calamity,
> And reaps a harvest-home of sorrow.'

Aeschylus (*The Persians*, 441 BC)

No patient should ever die because of ill-informed arrogance. I have seen rule-abiding doctors arrogantly apply regulations to a patient's management, when obviously not in the patient's best interest.

Attached and Detached

This applies most to doctors. Whereas scientists can readily understand humanitarian concepts (although not necessarily the subtleties), few who studied humanities understand much of science. There are doctors whose primary approach to patients is scientific, 'detached' and anonymous, and those whose approach is 'attached' and humanitarian. Both approaches produce results, but in ways not always acceptable to patients.

Patients need medical science, but once a person becomes a patient, it is usually those doctors and nurses with a talent for the art of medicine who they will welcome most. There are reasons for this which apply to every art. Unlike the transitive purposeful process of training to achieve distinct clinical objectives, the art of medicine embraces the intransitive. It requires us to use our sense of being. There need be no particular end-point in mind, other than patient satisfaction.

Read more in my book, *The Art and Science of Medicine*.

Autistic

To contact doctors on the autistic spectrum can be like accessing a computer avatar; a relationship that lacks true human responsiveness, empathy, or any appreciation of the plight of others (although one can train them to simulate it). Their approach to life is usually objective, mechanical, and algorithmic. They often enjoy categorising and struggle with all forms of interpersonal contact. They most enjoy being logical and self-oriented. They operate in a diplomacy-free world of their own, and make judgements derived from objective analysis, rather than any personal consideration. Their relationships and their decision-making processes can seem scripted. The art of medicine eludes them. With no need for human understanding, they can limit their considerations and suggestions to only those for which there is good evidence. If they were artists, they might choose to paint in black and white, rather than in colour.

Martin Clunes in the UK, TV series (2004-2009) '*Doc Martin*', the creation of Dominic Minghella, gives a perfect representation of an autistic doctor.

Bombast

These are self-assured doctors who deride almost everything suggested by others. With an air of 'knowing it all', their aim is to override anyone who dares not to share their view. They will counter every criticism with a well-rehearsed journal reference, or a quote from an unimpeachable source. At ward rounds, their aim is to make an impression, and to leave no-one in doubt of their cleverness and superior knowledge.

When I was a student, one of my lecturers at 'the London' would surreptitiously research all the cases to be presented at each weekly case conference. We were often astonished by his astute diagnoses. He made successful diagnoses using only one or two seemingly insignificant pieces of clinical information.

I met him many times later in life. Although he remained a clinical bombast, he was a very competent physician.

BBC: Baked **B**ean **C**ounter

*It is more important to make what is important mea-
surable, than to make what is measurable important.*

Simon Jenkins.

Data, rather than patient welfare, may consume the obsessional interest of these doctors and nurses. They prefer
calculation to caring; following orders, in preference to
deciding for themselves. They may have missed out on
their ideal profession – accountancy, or laboratory science.
These doctors are at their best, away from the bedside.
Many make successful PhD students, and some should
undertake yet further doctorate degrees, just to keep them
off the wards. They are important 'back-room boys', and
make valuable members of an academic team.

The bean counter's virtues are analytic. Their analyses
can help us avoid fooling ourselves. Competent doctors
will be pleased to have their management assessed once
all the clinical events have played out. Some clinicians
might then say, 'I could have told you so.' Such can be
the predictive power of long-acquired practical experience.
Data-driven bean-counters will often regard anecdote as
hearsay, and devoid of scientific value.

Hindsight is an exact science.

How would you spot a BBC if you have never met one
before? I recommend the Boulting brothers', 1959 comedy film, *'I'm All Right Jack'* (Charter Film Productions),

in which Peter Sellers plays Fred Kite. Fred is a Union official with stereotypical, measured speech; a typical bean counter.

Bean counters are usually serious, obsessional, and self-controlled. The Nazi SS officer Herr Otto Flick, played by Richard Gibson in the original TV series 'Allo, Allo', demonstrated the BBC character perfectly. Herr Flick delivers his carefully chosen words precisely. His speech has a commanding manner, delivered as if a metronome had set its pace. He kept any variation of speech rhythm to a minimum.

Do these doctors and nurses have a restricted, black and white character, rather than the full Technicolor version? Patients come to regard BBCs as unapproachable, unfriendly, and with limited communication skills. Some have a professional problem with intimacy and friendliness, but with a private persona that may differ from their public one.

Because they devote themselves to accuracy, they are ready to criticise, find fault, and correct others who do not accept their analyses. They often ask others to define what they mean.

Many see no need to endear themselves to patients. They are at their happiest in a totally controlled environment (preferably controlled by themselves), like a laboratory or operating theatre. They occasionally escape onto the wards where carers may choose to avoid them. Patients, unfortunately, will not escape them so easily.

I have happily collaborated with many BBCs and have occasionally been in BBC mode myself As a research fellow at St. George's Hospital, London, Aubrey Leatham regarded me as a 'back-room boy'. He dubbed me the cardiac department's 'man of fast cars, and slow rhythms'. He had seen me driving my yellow Lotus Elan 2+2 in the 1970s, while researching blackouts.

Mastery of any subject requires an extensive knowledge of the known and unknown. Experience and perspective will guide every master in any field, but bean counters are likely to view any clinical success derived from experience as 'luck'; they rarely believe in the usefulness of anecdote.

See also: 'Obsessives, and Nit-Pickers.' These present as perfectionist, so called 'anal' sub-groups, with no autistic element.

Bias Unaware People

All decision making is subject to bias. When making any evaluation or decision, one should consider the many cognitive biases outlined by Kahneman and Tversky in the 1970s. Every doctor needs to be aware of their biases and how they might influence their clinical judgement and decision making.

Big Picture Thinkers

There are undoubtedly those doctors who think big. They have their eye only on the top jobs. Like Winston Churchill, many have the premonition that, one day, greatness will strike.

In research terms, they know what is best to pursue. They will place themselves at the forefront of groundbreaking research. They often see the value of a subject, others are late to recognise. Recognising the growing need for shopping convenience, Jeff Bezos invented Amazon. He also suggested the need for rapid postal delivery services to save the time needed to search retail outlets.

Blackmailers

It is not entirely unknown for doctors, nurses, and other medical professionals to emphasise the negative consequences of not complying with their wishes. Some accept tacit threat as allowable professional manoeuvring, soft bullying, or gentle coercion; others call this blackmail.

Bores

Usually serious, often with a depleted sense of humour and a limited range of topics to interest others, these characters abound in the medical profession.

Bullies

Many newly qualified doctors feel vulnerable. Because their progress can depend on the impression they make, they might not react wisely to bullying. Bullies like to find a weak spot and continue to irritate it. Some senior doctors are intellectual bullies; they will out-quote their juniors in matters of medical science, in order to demean them. They will then dismiss them by quickly changing the subject.

In a survey of 416 junior doctors(in Europe-wide microbiology and infectious diseases), 22% reported bullying at work. Two-thirds also felt worn out, having had to work longer hours than normal .
Maraolo et al. 2017.

Carriers

In life terms, these are important people to identify. They arethemetaphorical geese capable of laying golden eggs. They appear to succeed in everything they do. Doctors and nurses should latch on to them (unless one themselves). Doctors should learn from them, perhaps by becoming their apprentice. They will make waves that are worth riding. They are going places.

My partner, Dr. David Baxter, was one such person. An extremely successful, energetic person, he enabled the development of our own private clinic in the 1973. His determination, energy, and ability made our success a foregone conclusion. After we parted, he continued to succeed and developed his own private hospital.

All such people are non-conformists. They are individuals, not groupies; shepherds, not sheep. Aspiring doctors and nurses will need to be compatible with these traits and brave enough to fly alongside them.

Capricious Creatures

Capricious doctors and nurses can find themselves bound into cycles of indecision and unnecessary repetition. One of my bosses always read my draft research papers many times before publication. If he didn't like it much, he would suggest alterations. After re-writing it, he would make further suggestions which returned it to the original text. One way of handling such people is to do very little. Their minds eventually tire of making half-hearted suggestions. Left alone to think it through, they might realise that their original suggestions were unhelpful.

Charming

Once a most desirable trait, but now not so common among doctors. Nurses more frequently possess it. Beware! In its false form, it sometimes combines with utter ruthlessness.

Club Members

In 1972, I was lucky enough to have a mentor for my Royal College of Physicians membership examination (MRCP). He pointed out that passing the examination was contingent on being 'the right sort of chap'. Perhaps this applies less now than it once did, but in the 1970s, passing the exam was not just a matter of knowing lots of medical facts. Then, it was as much to do with how doctors presented themselves to the examiners (Fellows of the Royal College of Physicians).

I came before three senior physicians, after reviewing a patient with complicated heart valve disease. They asked me to describe the heart sounds. This I did to the standard expected by Dr. Aubrey Leatham, then a world expert on heart sounds. They listened to me in silence, then asked, 'For whom do you work?' Then, 'How is Aubrey these days? Does he still walk between the Heart Hospital, and St. Georges every day (1.5 miles)? Does he still sail at West Wittering?' They had obviously accepted me as a member of their club.

Cold Fish

Emotionally deprived. Not unlike talking to a dead fish.

Combustible Consultants

Modelled on the cinema character Sir Lancelot Pratt (played by James Robertson Justice in *Doctor at Large*, Rank Film Distributors, 1957), some doctors can explode emotionally when annoyed.

My medical student friend, Leslie Dobson and I, used to attend the London University Wine Tasting Club every week. We rarely limited ourselves to sips of wine. Les became a connoisseur. The day after one such session, neither of us felt too well. Les had to assist a thoracic surgeon, well-known for his irascibility. I remained at a safe distance in the viewing gallery of the operating theatre. Les had turned slightly green and felt nauseated, while trying his best to assist the surgeon.

It was going to be a bad day. While trying to put on his surgical gloves, the surgeon asked Les how he was feeling (having noted the similarity of his facial colour to the green coloured surgical gowns we then wore). 'Not too good', he replied, understating the case. 'Well, pull yourself together, boy!', the surgeon suggested.

Something rare then happened. A nurse gave the surgeon a packet containing two left gloves. This caused him to show his irritation, and to shout a complaint. Nurses scrabbled around, hither and thither, in order to remedy the situation. They brought him another new packet. He tried on the second pair, only to find the same thing: two left gloves! The temperature in the operating theatre rose sharply. At this moment, Leslie had to admit that he felt ill, faint, nauseous, and about to vomit. The surgeon at once burst into an incandescent rage. A sympathetic nurse whisked Les away to vomit. A sympathetic senior theatre sister did her best to placate the surgeon and the situation. Fortunately, a normal pair of gloves soon arrived and everyone, including the patient, survived the experience.

My much respected, and greatly missed friend Dr. Leslie P. Dobson, served his North Yorkshire community as a GP for most of his working life. He died on the 2nd of March 2020.

Completer Finishers

Effective executive functioning is crucial for both doctors and nurses. Competent doctors can draw all the technical ends together, loose and otherwise, make a diagnosis and correctly decide on the most effective management. Those unable to do this in a co-ordinated way may need to revisit the same problem several times. They will see patients repeatedly and sometimes leave them with unanswered, worrying questions. The number of different diagnoses they generate can be a measure of their indecisiveness. The patient, meanwhile, will remain in suspense. This is behaviour for doctors and patients should avoid. Doctors should observe efficient, completer-finishers, and learn from them.

Control Freaks

These doctors and nurses are obsessive neurotics. They can be aggressive and uncompromising. King Canute remained unsure of why he wanted to control the tides, but then, not all control freaks seek reasons for what they do. Some are would-be puppeteers, others are shepherds. Either way, their concern is to take the reins and control others. They are usually selfish and want their way regardless of any cost to others.

There are reasons some doctors want control. Gaining power and recognition are among them. One method they use involves meticulous data collection and categorisation. They understand that information can be a powerful weapon. Some are harmless, like librarians; a few use information for malign purposes.

That information is power is hardly a new idea. The Ancient Egyptians collected personal information to enable taxation. The information in the Doomsday Book served the same purpose. Those people and organisations who collect personal information have many and various motives, some of them Machiavellian.

Cool Dudes

A few cool dudes are doctors and nurses. Love 'em or hate 'em, they remain cool in all circumstances. Study 'Cool.' The Complete Handbook, by Harry Armfield (1986), and consider fictional characters like Sean Connery's James Bond, or Winkler's character Fonzie (A. H. Fonzarelli). Few doctors are Fonzie-like; narcissistic peacocks who are constantly preening themselves. Some ooze pheromones, as they delight in themselves. The élite French recognise some as *BCBG: bon chic, bon genre*. Being cool and phlegmatic can be inborn, although some will try to learn how. They will not easily escape recognition by any true BCBG. There are questionnaires that rate 'cool', but no cool dude would ever begin or complete one.

Corporate Kids

These guys are at home in a corporate environment, fenced in by what they feel to be comforting rules and regulations. They try not to be controversial, undiplomatic, political, or anti-establishmentarian. If they keep their heads down, work hard, and do what others ask of them, their careers (and pensions) should flourish. Since the NHS is run as a corporation, the same will apply to many UK doctors and nurses.

DOD: Daft Old Doctors (or SOS, or Silly Old Sods)

When I first met the very experienced general surgeon, Mr. Douglas Lang-Stevenson (1912 – 1986), at Whipp's Cross Hospital, he was about to retire. He told me that 'stress caused cancer.' It sounded daft. Many thought him past his best. With decades of observation behind him, he deserved more respect. I have little to add, having seen too few cancer cases as a cardiologist, but it is still a worthy topic for research.

Having nothing to lose, the retired and those who are wealthy can be as daft and despotic as they like. Old doctors, like me, can be cogent pussy cats or dis-inhibited tigers. After decades of experience and being on the brink of dementia, it becomes easier to fool oneself. When old, we are liable to dream up a theory and stick to it, rather than bother to confirm it with extensive research and evidence. We can become less bothered about hard evidence and statistical likelihood, and more comfortable with the richer anecdotal evidence we have derived from experience.

Beware, though, some correct ideas sounded daft at first. Prestigious older scientists are liable to the same folly, despite their track record. Beware of adopting the halo bias in their presence. Like pop-singers, they may only be as good as their last hit.

After winning two Nobel Prizes, Linus Pauling proclaimed two theories. First, that vitamin C could prevent cancer, and second, that it would prevent heart attacks. In 1973, he established an institute in Oregon, partly to research his theories. Convincing confirmatory evidence for either hypothesis is still awaited. Theories are cheap, proof is expensive.

Older doctors do not always quick to accept innovation. When I asked a contemporary of mine from medical school to repair my umbilical hernia, he told me he didn't believe in using 'meshes'. He preferred the tried and trusted method of suturing (with the equivalent of football shoelaces). After a quick internet search that revealed a lower recurrence rate with meshes, I changed surgeons.

Daft ideas are not the sole preserve of the old.

When a patient of mine needed a pacemaker, the young professor of cardiology dealing with him (who was collecting cases for a trial), announced that he did not believe in 'implanting unnecessary bits of metal and plastic'. Was that enough justification for failing to pace a patient with a very slow heart rate and a history of sudden blackouts? Sudden blackouts can kill. Fifty years spent developing 'metal and plastic' of pacemakers has proven their safety.

PostScript: after one further blackout, which he was lucky to survive, the patient had a pacemaker implanted. That put an end to his symptoms and improved his well-being.

Dedicated Doctors and Nurses

I have encountered many dedicated doctors and nurses in my time and been honoured to work with them. Typically, they will selflessly support you, the system they work for, and their patients. They can be academics, hospital doctors, or GPs. Whatever their position in the profession, they are worthy of admiration and support for their humility and public service.

I would like to pay homage to one such doctor. He was once an NHS GP with a practice in Leytonstone, London. I met him a few times while working at Whipp's Cross Hospital in the late 1960s.

Irishman, Dr. Swift Daly, drove a large Humber Super Snipe in which he conveyed his sick patients to and from the 'Casualty', at Whipp's Cross Hospital (the term 'A&E' had yet to be used). He would sometimes arrive half-drunk with a sick patient in tow, leaving his other patients waiting for him at his surgery; these patients happily awaited his return. He once said to me, 'This patient isn't well. You're a nice young chap (a little blarney goes a long way). I am sure you will find out what's wrong with him. I'll wait outside while you examine him.' Afterwards, he would drive the patient back to his surgery, where he would continue with his other consultations. Those who took no time to get to know him thought he was a bit of a joke.

The police knew him well, and often escorted him to the hospital (at a time before any drink / driving laws). One of them told me he drank whisky during his consultations and then threw the empty bottles out into his garden. 'His garden is a sea of whisky bottles', one informed me.

I came to respect Dr. Swift-Daly's clinical acumen and wisdom. He was realistic and honest enough to know what he didn't know. Such characters did a lot for the profession by providing a selfless, dedicated service. For patients, his service transcended personal considerations. His patients undoubtedly respected and cared for him. I am confident that thousands of his loyal patients would acknowledge a debt to him.

Had the Care Quality Commission (CQC) then existed, I doubt they would have found his practice compliant. Would they have closed his practice and withdrawn his attentive services from hundreds of patients? Because their focus is now on potential risks, and not what is most valuable to patients, they would undoubtedly have checked many irrelevant boxes, and taken a negative view. Some regard what they do as progress. I doubt respected doctors, like Swift Daly and his patients, would have agreed.

Diagnostniks

The principle fulfilment of these doctors comes from making challenging diagnoses. Some enjoy the accolade of colleagues more than helping patients.

Dismissers

Whatever is suggested, this doctor will reject it, counter it, and dismiss it. Their opinion *is* the only one they value. Other doctors must know their arguments well and only counter them after thorough research. One can ambush them and defeat them by planning the attack. Although they are usually arrogant and best avoided, they may deserve respect for the contributions they once made. Being correct once gives them no right to think they will always be so.

Disrespectful

Most doctors I met during my career were respectful of the ideas of others, whatever their educational background, socio-economic standing, profession, or culture. Very few doctors were racist, with no interest in the culture or religion of their patients. Meanwhile, UK multi-racial demography marches on and their position is no longer tenable.

Disrespect can have intellectual origins. Seeing themselves as custodians of knowledge and intellect, educated, clever people can look down on the poorly educated. Some are sanctimonious and arrogant, and claim intellectual justification for the disrespect they have. One can easily find published examples of intentional intellectual disrespect. In Richard Dawkins' 'Outgrowing God', and 'The God Delusion', or Salman Rushdie's 'The Satanic Verses', disrespect for the beliefs of others obvious. In their pursuit of truth, the use of fiction, logical argument and parody can leave many feeling wounded and angry.

Doctors in high academic office can afford to disrespect the findings of their clinical and research colleagues. Those who disrespect patients will usually remove themselves from (the menial task of) having to deal with them.

DPSWs: Dedicated **P**ublic **S**ector **W**orkers.

Some doctors and nurses work in public services. Some are to be found managing the NHS. Because they decide what services doctors and nurses can give, many feel they occupy the moral high ground. Some view their work in public services as 'worthy', and medical services as 'unworthy', although they might change their view, once they acknowledge that the NHS can no longer cope.

Over the course of my career, I have known many DPSWs who despised the private sector. Some would not bring themselves to acknowledge any benefit in having private hospitals or private medical facilities. They must have found it challenging to know that captains of industry, company directors, the self-employed, government ministers, and the Royal Family, prefer private medical services. Some may not be so ready to acknowledge why, given a little embarrassment about long NHS waiting times, NHS queues for admission, and NHS bed shortages. Their sanctimony and biases may have to change as they off-load NHS 'cold-cases' to private sector hospitals. Private practices now lessen the burden on the NHS, but this too they may choose not to acknowledgement.

Believing public services to be superior in every way, some still voice the opinion that 'Patients would be mad to pay when the NHS is free.'

DAS: Doctors As Scoundrels

You might think that less than honourable behaviour is to be found only among politicians, second-hand car dealers and criminals, but not doctors or nurses. You would be wrong. Some doctors will steal the ideas and secrets of others, and are readily capable of skulduggery, cheating, dishonesty, sycophancy, spying, back stabbing, jealousy, avarice, and vindictiveness. I have experienced them all, and have detected most of them early enough to avoid the consequences.

I was born into a business family and exposed to 'street wisdom' from an early age. I grew up learning to avoid advantage-takers, but did not expect to find them among my professional colleagues. For a life in medical practice, should one really have to study Machiavellian tactics?

A GP I worked with always did lots of home visits, or so we thought. He registered them every day in our practice work diary and visited patients after 'surgery' hours. We all admired him for making 5 to 10 home visits every day. That was until one of my smarter colleagues checked on him. He telephoned his patients to ask when last a doctor visited them. Surprise, surprise. The doctor in question had visited very few.

Later on, at the same practice, I found out that we juniors were paying for two extra doctors attached to the practice. Their wages and expenses were being deducted from our salaries, not from those of the senior partners. Their argument, when discovered, was that we juniors were the ones who needed help. My argument was that they helped us all. I won the day by enquiring into their other, less than scrupulous ac-

counting practises, and by asking, 'Are the Inland Revenue aware of what you are doing?'

All very unpleasant. To discover doctors playing dirty tricks can be disappointing. Being naïve can be endearing, but it comes with disadvantages.

Some doctors are devious, and just as likely to pursue skulduggery for personal gain, as anyone else. When Dorothy walked along the yellow brick road in the Land of Oz, she did so with loyal friends. Many doctors and nurses progress in the medical profession, accompanied by tigers, lions, and bears and others who do not always have their best interests at heart.

It is easy to steal ideas. Since I have always been inventive, I have generated more research ideas than I have had time to develop. For those who lack ideas, it could be expedient to steal some, in order to progress their career. This has happened to me several times.

'Where do you get your ideas from, Victoria?
'I don't know. But, if I ever find out, I'm going to live there.'
Victoria Wood.

While I was still practising, I had an enterprising (entrepreneurial) group of doctors try to gain access to my practice information. They were asking too many questions, with no obvious intent to collaborate. 'What's in it for them?' I wondered. I guessed they were after my database of patients and my methods of working. Doctors, like me, who have survived for so long in independent private practice, hold valuable information. The benefits of experience are invaluable and easily stolen.

Ideas make money, and for doctors born into a business culture, there is a rule - it is easier and cheaper to copy the work of others, than to create anew. What these doctors will not have appreciated is that there is no shortcut to building a lasting medical practice. Gaining the confidence of smart, successful patients takes time. My guess is that they wanted something different - to franchise private GP services. Their objectives may have represented the sunny slopes of capitalism, but for me, they represented the shady side of commercialised medicine.

Not long after visiting me, these doctors copied my prepayment medical scheme (created by me in 1985) and promoted it on their website. This was not my original idea. I modelled it on American HMO schemes. It became much appreciated by my less wealthy patients, and remained unchallenged, or copied, for 35-years.

Another common form of scoundrel is 'the user'. I am sad to say that among the many doctors I have met, I found just as many 'users' as in other walks of life. Doctors and nurses need to be aware of sweet-talking, less capable colleagues, whose aim is to get their work done for them. For some, it is their natural inclination. For less sinister characters, it may simply be a matter of laziness or convenient delegation.

My suggestion to doctors is to work only with those who are secure and mature enough, not to need to steal ideas. Such people would sooner promote you than use you. You may think that sounds paranoid. After being exposed to it, some doctors may think differently.

Many of those 'at the top' of any profession will have trodden on others on the way up to their prestigious pinnacle of power. Under the Peter Principle, many of them will have arrived at their level of incompetence. Doctors and nurses must know that power-seekers, thieves, users, and the avaricious, abound in all walks of life. Among them will be medical colleagues.

Dork

Those with two left feet may be born inept; some become valuable techno-geeks. Awkward, and sometimes socially inadequate, there are plenty of them in the medical profession. They can be endearingly eccentric and make valuable contributions.

Egoists

You will not have to wait long before you meet your first egoist colleague. They have strong opinions which they will usually broadcast forcefully. Not all are bigots. Some are 'Jumpers': jumping quickly to a conclusion, and moving on in order to end any further reasoned discussion. The implication is, 'I know best, so let's not tarry'. Those with the experience and the evidence-base at their fingertips deserve respect, but doctors should never let their ego suppress independent critical thought.

Emotionally Unfit

The intellectual ability needed to pass medical examinations is no guide to a doctor's ability to cope with emotionally laden situations. Given problems at home and stress at work, they may not cope at all well emotionally. There were a few among my medical student colleagues, and I encountered a few more as a junior doctor. In the old days, colleagues would have stepped in and helped. Not all recovered sufficiently to re-consider continuing their medical career. Prince Harry and Prince William deserve the congratulations they received for exposing long-suppressed mental health issues.

Michael Palin on his 'Full Circle' trip of the world (BBC ONE, 1997) came across the grave of Commander Stokes. Pringle Stokes was captain of HMS Beagle on its first voyage around South America. Inscribed on his memorial cross (12.8.1828) is, 'he died from the effects of the anxieties and hardships incurred while surveying the western shores of Tierra del Fuego.' The result was that he committed suicide. Charles Darwin was on the second voyage of the Beagle (1831-6).

ERP: Emotionally Reactive People

Such doctors and nurses are quick to 'throw their toys out of their cot' when not getting what they want. With weak parents, they would have successfully used this behaviour as a child. Some will continue to do so when they sense they are close to their competence limit; others will not give up trying it, just to get instant gratification. They are best avoided, except to offer them psychotherapy.

The aetiology of such reactivity is often simple. As children, nobody reprimanded them, and they behaved as they wished. Those too weak to resist their tantrums spoiled them; perhaps fearing the loss of their affection. Throwing tantrums got them what they wanted, so they continued with the same unacceptable behaviour into adulthood. They may not yet have met someone willing to stand up to them, but they will. Some are underdeveloped emotionally. My advice is for doctors and nurses to recognise them, and move away as fast as possible. Those who choose to remain in their orbit may hope to change them, claiming them to be misunderstood.

Favorites

There are many reasons for a senior to see a junior doctor or nurse as 'the chosen one'; prized just a little more than seems appropriate. The reason for such favouritism is sometimes unclear. The blindness of uncritical admiration or the star-struck effect of beauty, wealth, and fame are real, but all based on 'fantasy'. My advice to third party onlookers is not to get involved.

There is a quieter, longer-term strategy to consider for the colleagues of favoured ones. Play it like Stalin during the Russian Revolution. He took a back seat and waited for the adored ones (Trotsky and Lenin) to fall from grace. He then stepped in and took over.

Flirts and Flatterers

'Flattery will get you everywhere.'

Mae West, Actress

Very few doctors, nurses, and patients are averse to being flattered, although few will find flatterers as overt as the eyelash fluttering Miss Piggy, in her quest to seduce Kermit the Muppet (TV series, ABC Studios). There are other amusing examples, like the girl dragon in the film *Shrek* (Universal Pictures, 2001). She effectively endears Donkey with her loving, dreamy-eyed eyelash fluttering. In a more subtle way, criminally flirtatious Wanda (Miss Wanda Gershwitz, played by Jamie Lee Curtis) in the film *A Fish Called Wanda*), gets her wicked way with the formal

British barrister, Archie Leach (Cary Grant's birth name), played by John Cleese. If you want to see flattery at work, watch these films.

Persuasion is especially effective when an attractive seducer unexpectedly shows an interest in one not so attractive. Some complement beautiful creatures, falsely claiming to have recognised their superior intelligence. It is surprising how much capacity some have to swallow compliments. Flatterers know this, and will escalate their compliments to the limit of acceptability (often to the astonishment of onlookers).

'What do you want?', and, 'What's in it for me?', are the key questions for those being flattered. Succumbing to flattery rarely leads to satisfaction. The best thing is to play flatterers at their own game, and understand their motives. If you call their bluff, you might become an adversary; the more attractive or important they are, the less prepared they are for rejection.

Frustrated Doctors and Nurses

NHS work conditions have angered and frustrated many doctors and nurses. Some have become disheartened and demoralised. They expect to fly like eagles and instead find themselves grounded like turkeys. Unrequited expectation is a powerful force for resentment. It can depress mood, reverse a positive outlook, and limit motivation.

Highly intelligent people can find it frustrating to deal with the uneducated, some of whom have searched the Internet, and want to dictate their needs to doctors. These encounters are potential sources of frustration and disappointment.

Fumblers

Whether it is putting up intravenous drips, taking blood, or examining patients, some doctors and nurses are downright awkward, seeming to fumble over every practical task. The doctors among them will not make talented surgeons. Hopefully, few will attempt to become one.

As an anaesthetist for one year, I had the chance to observe many surgeons at work. What surprised me was the variability of their co-ordination and mechanical dexterity.

GAHAD: Good At Hiding All Deficiencies

In some cultures, not to lose face has a higher priority than telling the truth. Whatever their culture, there are some who will always try to cover-up their shortcomings. If a doctor or nurse ever injects the wrong drug or wrongly performs a procedure, they must declare it immediately. Using the principle of 'patients first', every medical team should help to correct the mistake. The patient's interest is never best served by a cover-up. Patients can die, and the perpetrators barred from practice.

A doctor or nurse will need bravery to become a whistle-blower. Up to now, many whistle-blowers have paid a high price for their revelations. There is a worrying lesson to be learned here: doctors and nurses should never expect their colleagues, members of management or regulators to support them. Many will want to save themselves from admonishment by disassociating themselves from whistle-blowers and those under investigation by the GMC.

Julius Caesar was not the last to be shocked by the betrayal of all his friends.

Glory Seekers

Has the need for glory changed over the centuries?

In Xenophon's dialogue *Ieron (Hiero)*, written in the 4th century BC., it says that all humans are free to enjoy food, sex, and drink, but only superior beings lust for honour, distinction and glory.

'But they in whom is implanted a passion for honour and praise, these are they who differ most from the beasts of the field, these are accounted men and not mere human beings.'

Ieron. (Chapter 7, section 3). Xenophon.

Hobbes, in *The Leviathan* (1651), states that the attainment of glory (as a means of recognition), with competition (for gain), and diffidence (for protection), are all strong motivating factors. Together they cause quarrels. Competitiveness and a desire for glory are not uncommon traits among doctors and nurses.

For doctors, glory will come only rarely, and be mostly limited to those who publish 'game-changing' research. Some will attain a lesser form of glory in public office, but gaining a knighthood, or peerage, will take a lot of nodding agreement, networking, and avoidance of conflict.

The focus of some doctors is not clinical at all. Their aim is to make their mark as regulators, NHS executives, or as politicians. For them, studying medicine is but a stepping stone.

GGs: Good Guys

Many good people can be found among patients, nurses, and doctors. There are many pleasant, fair, respectful, diplomatic and reasonable people around. They have grace and charm as virtues. They will display 'good behaviour' at all times, and resist corruption by NBW's (Nasty Bits of Work, see later). Good behaviour is easy to define. It is that which leaves everyone feeling comfortable. Sadly, the opposite is ubiquitous. 'Good Guys' are usually obvious from the first moment you meet them. Time will not change your impression. I have only met a few in my lifetime.

Gossips ('Newsmongers', according to Theophrastus)

Gossips are everywhere in hospitals and medical practices. Some wish to convey only light-hearted hearsay; others can be sinister, hateful, and derogatory.Often the subject is, 'who is screwing whom?' Gossip gains in interest with its level of secrecy.

The Biblical crime of a loose or evil tongue (defamation), as committed by Miriam, can damage three people: the one who propagates it, the person it concerns, and the one who listens. It seems rather harsh to accept that it is worse than idolatry, incest, and murder, but that was the Biblical view (Dr. Jonathon Sacks, former UK Chief Rabbi, *The Power of Praise*, 2018).

Grammar School versus Public School

Doctors and nurses typically receive education from grammar and public schools. Grammar school alumnae and alumni are typically intelligent and well informed. Their tendency is to be self-righteous. As insecure socialists, many are outspoken, attention seeking, brusque, and aspire to utopian ideals.

Michael Portillo observed, in a BBC Four programme about Grammar Schools, that Public School boys had more effortless charm and confidence. Because of financial pre-selection, British public school pupils are usually more secure. They less often display an intense demeanour and mostly show quiet respect for their peers. These are the result of being banged up in a boarding school for years. Many have the unfortunate tendency to side-line those from lower socio-economic backgrounds, but they will leave fewer rattled by their behaviour than their Grammar school contemporaries. Because those who we find most attractive usually come from our own social group, our class-ridden UK society remains steadfast.

It may be out-of-date, but for those working in the major professions: medicine, the Church, and the law, public school characteristics remain *de rigueur* for candidate selection in the UK. The last decade has seen moves to make more places in public schools and Oxbridge for the less privileged, but in reality, there are too many levels of conflict for this to be a comfortable experience for those involved.

Gunslinger

This type of doctor is rare. A colleague of mine was one. He was both aggressive and uncompromising, and once wrote to a patient telling him he would be 'mad not to comply' with his advice. He followed this with, 'Why die for the sake of having one straightforward operation?' He said he had no time for 'stupid people', and often suggested that such patients should find another doctor. His policy was to 'take no prisoners', and to challenge problems head on; both features helped him to succeed in life.

His private consultant colleagues once approached him about his behaviour and management style while running his own private hospital. They threatened to get him 'struck-off' of the GMC register. His reply was: 'Since I own this hospital, I can employ as many consultants like you as I like. Don't waste my time with idle threats.' They crept away with their tails between their legs. My advice is not to engage a professional gunslinger without a lot of prior shooting practice. Doctors and nurses need to remember not to box above their weight!

Haughty

Nose in the air, self-possessed, and consumed with their self-importance, some doctors (and to a much lesser extent nurses) will treat most others as lesser beings. This is not an uncommon trait.

Hero, Champion and Role Model

All doctors and nurses will have identified fellow pupils, teachers, or colleagues, who they admire for their knowledge, wisdom, helpfulness, and effectiveness. Hopefully, they will inspire the same reverence someday.

I am sad to say that as a lecturer for seven years, I remember only a few of my students. I taught many, however, who remember me. For any teacher to achieve this status is a worthy achievement. Doctors must not expect this to count in their favour if they ever get entangled with the CQC or the GMC. With the statutory power they brandish, some now believe their value to society to be greater than any doctor or nurse.

High-Minded

'Glory is my object, and that alone.'

Horatio Lord Nelson.

Nelson's sentiment will ring true for a few doctors. There are plenty who crave the Presidency of their Royal College, or a royal appointment. They are always a little coy about declaring it.

Many authors have known such doctors. George Eliot, author of *Middlemarch* (1871), mentions the ambitious, but tragic, Dr. Lydgate. His ambitions were to pursue research and treat fevers in a novel way, according to the latest French theories. Not all authors have portrayed doctors in a good light. Both Chaucer and Shakespeare saw doctors as money grabbing, and low-minded (not an entirely unfounded view of the occasional doctor to-day).

Hobby Horse Enthusiasts

Beware of fixated doctors. They will try to explain every condition in terms of their particular hobby horse interest. (See 'Spanophilia').

Mr. Bill K. was an anxious hypochondriac. A highly specialised cardiac research team mapped his cardiac disease (amyloid). In consultation with him, they described his problem in worrying detail. The studies were of academic interest, but that is not how the patient came to view them. He came to see me, to ask what I thought.

My echocardiograms had revealed a slight problem, but then he was 85-years-old. My opinion was that his condition was of academic interest only, and unlikely to affect his life expectancy significantly.

Unfortunately, the harm was done. The repeated explanations of research enthusiasts, who found him to be 'an interesting case', emotionally destabilised Bill. He became depressed and withdrawn, the opposite of his more usual happy demeanour.

Enthusiastic, detached researchers, carried away by their interest in scientific detail, can ignore patient sensitivity. They presumably regard the science of medicine as more important to patients than the art of medicine.

Hobbyists

These are doctors whose hobby is medicine. They delight in meeting patients and everything medical fascinates them, especially interesting cases and the latest research. They have ceased to regard the practise of medicine as work, and feel privileged to get paid for pursuing their hobby.

There is a negative aspect to this. They can regard their work as a game, created just for their amusement. While enjoying their hobby, they may make light of how illness can affect patients. They make agreeable companions, and I have always found their enthusiasm for medicine infectious and edifying. We need more of them.

Hollow Men

T.S. Eliot referred to such people in his poem of the same title (1926), their eyes lacking life, spontaneity, and vigour, 'As the hollow men. The stuffed men ... The hope only of empty men.'

Some doctors and nurses become depressed, others have an insufficient interest in medicine and its practise.

Humorous Fellows

Although many doctors are capable of wit and a little innocent banter, many see humour as inappropriate and unprofessional when patients are present. Serious professionals have traditionally discouraged humour. As an advanced inter-personal technique for doctors and nurses, I cannot recommend it, even though it was my own USP. It will only attract those patients happy with the approach. It will offend others.

Seriousness does not always connote competence and expertise, and light-heartedness is not always frivolous. Humour can dispel anxiety and fear and can replace the face of impending doom with a smile. Humour can impart a message, but to use it requires talent and practice. Dr. Patch Adams' style provides a noteworthy example of its use, few are able to emulate.

A few doctors have become professional comics; the rest tempt providence when using humour during consultations. Unless doctors know their patient well, it can fall flat and embarrass. It is perfectly possible to be serious (and scientific) on one occasion, and humorous on another. The ability to judge which is appropriate is an art.

'Timing is everything', said Bob Hope, and this means choosing the right moment. The right remark, the witty aside, and a relevant joke, can inspire confidence and breakdown formality. Jokes can ruin a doctor-patient relationship when used facetiously, or when used in poor taste. One problem with humour is that some patients will be too preoccupied to appreciate it. For others, it can divert their introspection and dissolve their fear for a while.

My patient was in hospital, awaiting an urgent hysterectomy. She was losing a lot of blood. As I entered her room she looked pale and frightened. The nursing staff were rushing around, clearly tense and worried. They had imparted their sense of urgency to her and caused her more worry about her fate. 'Am I going to die, doctor?' she asked me. Because I knew her well, and knew she had a good sense of humour,

I replied, 'Not without my permission you're not!' It made light of a tense, high-risk situation. I followed that with, 'As a private doctor, I cannot afford to lose patients!' That made her smile, and she relaxed a little.

When I next saw her, she had survived a successful emergency hysterectomy. She thanked me for dispelling some of her fear and giving her some confidence. She said, 'When I knew you weren't worried, I relaxed. You helped me believe I was not about to die. Thank-you.'

When a patient acknowledges a doctor's humour, it will be obvious from their reaction. Humour shared, can leave both parties with a sense of 'us', rather than the usual 'you (doctor), me (patient)'. It can affirm mutual understanding. The further apart cultural values are between people, the less likely they are to share humorous moments. The risk is that humour will fall flat or offend, leaving both parties feeling alienated.

The late Mike Reid (Cockney actor and comedian), was once my patient. I had the temerity to tell him a joke. While consulting with him, he stood up, and without another word went straight to my receptionist and asked, 'Who is that guy? Is he a doctor, or a comedian? Doesn't he know that I'm the comedian here?'

Joking and making light of situations is typical of Cockney humour. Even the Luftwaffe failed to dampen it during the Blitz of London in the 2nd World War. My parents, grandparents, and all my great-grandparents were Cockneys (born within the sound of Bow bells, in the East End of

London), so Mike and I shared a culture which made our
understanding of one another an easy matter.

Idol or Idle?

Many of us come to idolise, or at least think well, of
the teachers who helped us most. They deserve it for
giving their pupils invaluable gifts: knowledge, understanding, and sometimes wisdom.

Some doctors and nurses will get bored with medicine and become idle. They may have chosen medicine as a career in order to satisfy family aspirations,
or simply wanted to gain status and security. Some will
know, right from the start, that their career choice was a
mistake, others will happily retire early. If demoralised
by 'the system' in which they work, some will disengage,
become idle and quit.

The demoralisation of many nurses and doctors working
in the NHS is now undoubted. Junior doctors are being
demoralised by a growing need to comply with manageri-
al interventions and corporate conventions, rather than to
be guided by their medical education, clinical experience
and judgement. It is now unwise for doctors to think for
themselves. Looking over their shoulder will be a manager
or regulator waiting to accuse them of non-compliance.

Jealous Creatures

Among both nurses and doctors, professional jealousy
is common. It can be the focus of many things – the talent of another doctor, physical attractiveness, popularity,
background, financial or class status, and reputation. The

ramifications can lead to trouble and a waste of time to deal with.

JGGs: Jolly Good Guys

These are very pleasant, honest, and amicable doctors and nurses. They make decent friends and are agreeable and sociable to work with. Some wear their superior knowledge and expertise lightly; others seem to know nothing at all. Supportive and pleasant to be around, they can make arduous work bearable. Those with a sense of humour can ease the burden of work with an anecdote or two, even while performing challenging tasks. Those easiest to associate with are those with no need to prove their talent. Doctors and nurses should look for amicable companions who have humility, and are generous and open enough to share the benefits of their talents.

Friedrich Nietzsche (Aphorisms on Love and Hate) had it that those who would be our friends are of two types: ladder and circle. The ladder types are going onward and upward. They will only be your friend as they pass you by. Others form circles; circles of friends you will keep for a lifetime.

Know It All

These are knowledgeable guys, likely to use information well, but sometimes to embarrass others. They can use their knowledge to shock or impress. Some can be monotonous, egotistical bores, strongly motivated to correct other people. Those who ask their opinion may need to reserve time for a lecture.

Lazy on Purpose

Doctors and nurses are not usually lazy, but should recognise those with laziness of a divisive kind. Laziness can be perversely attractive to those inclined to help others with their work. A lack of adroitness, alacrity, or panache will draw some to their rescue. Amid profuse thanks, some will seduce their helper into becoming their servant. They are good at flattery. They know that the more praise they give, the more vulnerable some become. Before they know it, some doctors will ask others to put up all their iv infusions, and perform all their routine tasks, while they put their feet up. I exaggerate, of course, but not as much as you might think.

The study of gamesmanship (author Stephen Potter) can help some to become successfully lazy. This is the basis of the film 'School for Scoundrels' (Associated British Picture Corp., 1960) with parts played by Terry Thomas, Ian Carmichael, and Alastair Sim. The film depicts the advantages of one-upmanship and gamesmanship. Like much good comedy, it explores serious, real-life relationships and shows how some can get the better of others. Techniques well worth studying for everyone wanting to gain control. Commonly found in medical professionals.

Legalist

The legalist is forever reminding others of the rules, regulations, and guidelines that apply in any situation. They are mostly obsessive and compulsive; baked-bean counters destined for bureaucracy or the chairmanship of committees.

Highly disciplined, dutiful, authoritarian types of nurse and doctor can be strict about adhering to all the accepted rules (as a matter of principle). The strict and punctilious sometimes dislike those who flout the rules, even when acting as needed.

The TV series 'Blackadder Goes Forth' portrays many clashes between an authoritarian and one who is dismissive of the rules. 'Darling' (Captain K. Darling), is a nit-picker, appropriately assigned to unloading and sorting paper-clips. He clashes with 'Blackadder', who cares little for bureaucratic rules, given the probability of his death as a front-line officer in the First World War.

There are military examples of similar clashes. The cunning, non-rule-based Viet-Cong in Vietnam defeated the US military repeatedly. This is partly because the US army has always been based on following strict rules of engagement. Such adherence helped to cause their demise. Al-Qaeda in Afghanistan inflicted a similar fate on the US army. General McCrystal, in his book *'Team of Teams'*, states that in the early days of US Army action in Afghanistan, they lacked the versatility of small terrorist groups. They had insufficient independent mindedness to change tactics as circumstances required.

Rules work best where predictability reigns, like running a bank or a railway network. Rule-based functioning cannot deal with some exceptions. Since exceptions are the stuff of medical practice, creative behaviour is more often valuable than stereotyped, rule-based behaviour. For this reason, doctors should only obey rules as 'guidelines', never as 'fixed' rules to be followed blindly. Our regulators do not agree. They can only regulate with fixed rules in place, so they commit medical intellectual heresy when they insist that doctors and nurses use guidelines as fixed immutable rules.

Little Sh*ts

These are doctors and nurses who will not mind dropping others in the sh*t, if it suits them. They are often self-possessed, arrogant, and superior. They can be short and dismissive of both patients and those of lower rank.

LMF (Lacking Moral Fibre)

Battle trauma was first recognised late during the First World War. Some military
personnel had 'battle fatigue', others had shell shock. Over two hundred soldiers accused of malingering, desertion and dereliction of duty were executed.

The British armed forces did not officially recognise post-traumatic syndrome (PTSD) until after the Falkland's war of 1982. The RAF, in particular, long referred to such cases as 'Lacking Moral Fibre.'

After qualification, some doctors will experience a few situations they find difficult to cope with. As such, they will struggle to make effective front-line interventionists. Given that many of the doctors who educated me served in the Second World War (WW2), the tacit accusation of LMF must have been on their minds when they witnessed a junior doctor failing to cope mentally with emergency situations. As a result, they would direct them to specialities like dermatology, general practice, and psychiatry, rather than interventional cardiology, A&E, and surgery. LMF is a completely unacceptable term, but like many others that are politically incorrect, they often contain more than a grain of truth.

Lone Wolf

Many doctors and nurses will work with anti-social, high achieving colleagues, some of whom will have Asperger features. There are doctors who belong in a world of their own; a world they rule alone. Fortunately, they will mostly choose to minimise their contact with colleagues and patients. (see: 'Doctors as Eccentrics'). Some are simply introverted and shy.

Lucky Buggers and the Matthew Effect

'For unto every one that hath shall be given, and shall have abundance: but from him that hath not shall be taken even that which he hath.'
                    Matthew 25:29. King James' Bible.

A junior doctor colleague of mine once experienced the 'Matthew' effect when on duty one night in 1966.

Junior doctor Tom was a rich Bahamian who shared alternate nights on duty with me. We were both first year housemen. The night he was on duty, he admitted an octogenarian lady with pneumonia. 'I have no family or heirs', she said. 'Would you agree to be my beneficiary?'

Tom eventually inherited 13 terraced houses, and £70,000 in cash (one could then buy a three-bed, terraced house in the area for £3000). His family owned a chain of hotels throughout the Bahamas, and my guess was that he had little need for any extra money. Money goes to money, they say. That's life!

Stand around a roulette table for long enough, or attend a horserace meeting or two, and you will see those who seem to win more than they lose. The majority do not win, of course, yet there are those who always fall on their feet, and those who always fall on their head.

Is having bad and good luck an illusion? There is a division of opinion about it. Chance will have it that unusually lucky people (those who beat the odds most of the time) must emerge, if given enough time. I remember one lucky doctor, selected for a prestigious job only because the interview board could not decide between the two more suitable candidates.

Amundsen, the polar explorer, did not rely on luck either. At the beginning of the 20th century, Roald Amundsen beat Scott to the South Pole. In fact, he was the first to reach both Poles. He wrote: 'Victory awaits him who has everything in order – luck, people call it. Defeat is certain for him who has neglected to take the precautions in time; this they call bad luck.'

A friend of mine deserved his luck. Nigel Nodolsky had generously given a kidney to someone he hardly knew. Because he became a research program subject he was regularly reviewed. A follow-up chest X-ray revealed a small lung lesion, which proved to be early lung cancer. No evidence of spread was found after its removal. This was good luck, but luck very much deserved because of Nigel's selfless generosity.

As an example of bad luck, my patient Oliver O'Rouke came to me with what proved to be a rare tonsillar cancer. Within one year, he returned with tongue cancer. The year after that, I diagnosed his prostate cancer. I regarded him as very unlucky. Because he was a JGG, he made light of it all. Sadly, he died in 2024.

Once I realised the gift of exceptional luck was not mine, I expected never to win anything by chance. I have stuck to what the American military once called: **PPPP: P**repara-tion **P**revents **P**oor **P**erformance, rather than luck (from the TV series M*A*S*H; 20th Century Fox Television). It has served me well.

Manipulators

For who would bear the whips and scorns of time,
Th'oppressor's wrong, the proud man's contumely,
The pangs of despised love, the law's delay,
The insolence of office . . .

Hamlet.
Act 3, Scene 1.

Unfortunately, doctors and nurses will only be posi-tioned to choose their colleagues once they achieve se-niority. Those who are 'manipulators', and 'controllers' by nature, will want to achieve this status as soon as possible. The naïve, the dedicated, and the altruistic don't usually give a damn about status; not until they have tasted the effects of manipulation. Their first reaction may then be: 'I didn't think doctors or nurses could be like that!'

The medical profession is replete with head-strong, arrogant egotists, who would give Niccolò Machiavelli a run for his money. Where survival and success are the issues, cunning and intelligence are both required for successful strategic planning. Cunning and a desire to manipulate others result from a predatory outlook. Both soon come to light in any relationship.

A common strategy used by predators is to keep secrets. The simple rule is: if you want to keep a secret (and avoid manipulation), tell nobody, and I mean – nobody.

Some health professionals are guilty of a minor confidence trick. Some osteopaths and dentists now call themselves 'doctors'. Will boosting their supposed status attract business and instil trust?

I once knew an ex-nurse who falsely purported to be a graduate doctor and psychiatrist. He was neither, although he did qualify as a psychiatric nurse. His wife, who came from the Far East, told her family that she had married an eminent doctor. This harmless folie a deux, suited them both.

'We schoolmasters must temper discretion with deceit.'

Dr. Fagan to Pennyfeather.*Decline and Fall* (1928).
Evelyn Waugh.

.

Phillipe was a suave, Gauloises smoking Lebanese doctor. He came to us as an observer in the cardiac department at Charing Cross Hospital, and constantly boasted about his family fortune: their multimillion dollar yacht moored in Monaco's Hercules harbour, and their villa on the Côte d'Azur. He also boasted that he was soon to open a smart medical Clinique, on Rue Cambon, Paris, alongside Chanel. It was to be equipped with the latest state-of-the-art medical equipment. Exaggeration, surely? He failed to manipulate us into thinking well of him.

Many years later, having not seen him for some time, I telephoned him from Amsterdam to say that I would soon be in Paris for a medical conference. He suggested we meet for lunch and view his medical facilities. We met for lunch, and he then showed me his clinic. It must have cost millions to put together. It was busy with patients drawn from the Parisian élites. Not all that seems hyperbole is a rhetorical confidence trick.

Beware of manipulators versed in *gamesmanship*; they can influence professional progress of doctors and nurses. Both the real and metaphorical chess players among us plan their moves well ahead of time, while non-gamers simply get on with the job of practising medicine. The gamer's short-term aim is to collect 'brownie points' from influential people; undoubtedly something they have done all their life. They will have employed stealth and even underhandedness to advance their career.

The aim of many manipulators is to attain high office. From that lofty position, they will have a strategic advantage over all challengers. They may then exhibit what Hamlet referred to as 'the insolence of office'. My advice is to identify them early, and side-step them quickly. If you don't, you may witness them walking away with prizes gained from manipulating colleagues. Another strategy would be to befriend them and become their second in command.

Doctors and nurses have all met one or two manipulators at school, or during their training. They must be prepared to meet some more when the stakes are higher. Hopefully, no doctor or nurse has to share their job with one. Those who do, might do all their work for them while they take all the credit. It is best not to share confidences with them. They will file these away for later use against you, at a time that suits their purpose. Learn to keep useful information secret until it benefits you. I would advise all doctors and nurses to keep their best cards up *their* sleeve, or close to *their* chest, and protect them from cunning predators and manipulators.

In order to prepare for such people, there is no better experience than attending a British independent public school. There, one will find those from successful backgrounds, some with family wealth funded on manipulation. There, one can learn their methods, and the earlier in life they are learned, the better. Contrast such people with doctors and nurses who simply love their job, and will do everything they can to help their colleagues and patients.

Controllers, manipulators and users will want to draw doctors and nurses into their circle. One must resist them, however tempting their inducements. Never risk becoming a puppet on their string.

I was once told that I was in line for a professorship . . . but there would be a price to pay. My response was immediate.
I doubted I could afford the price, whatever it was. The colleague who suggested it dismissed me with a compliment:
'You are too secure, Dighton', he said, realising that I under-

stood his attempted manipulation. The corporate life was not going to be for me.

Mean Bastards

The university medical degrees, MB., BS are not an acronym for **M**ean **B**astard, **B**latently **S**elfish, but they can be! Some doctors help only themselves. There have always been many of them.

Military

Ex-military personnel are easy to spot. They have a disciplined dress-sense, a respectful manner, highly polished shoes, and a noticeable personal bearing. Confident, dependable, and dutiful, they are usually reliable as doctors, nurses or patients.

Moralist

They are forever reminding others of the need for morality. Ethicists will remind us of the rules of engagement.

NAGS: 'Needs of A Good SH*G!'

Rarely uttered; often thought. This can be the most appropriate treatment for those who have become uptight and irritable. Sexual intercourse will usually calm their angst and make them more amenable (see 1980s TV mini-series *Shōgun*, Paramount TV. Original book by James Clavell). Studious types who have spent too long studying (rather than getting out, having a good time, and loosening up) will also benefit. We urgently need double-blind trials to verify the efficacy of this treatment.

Names

What's in a name? Doctors with unforgettable names, especially those that are double-barrelled, once progressed faster than others in the medical profession. If parents wanted their child to get on in the medical profession, they would name their boys Peregrine, Hugh, Sebastian, Tristram or Guy, and their girls Lucretia, Claudia, Tabatha, or Hermione. These names are not only striking to those in authority, but easily remembered. A distinguished name will not guarantee progress through the ranks, but it's a good start. Later on, they will be required to live up to the image their name projects.

Once highly respected were noble foreign surnames. Today, they can be regarded as pretentious. The French aristocratic name, Chalut de Bascoigne, rhymes with the name of one of my contemporaries at 'The London'. Once qualified, he rapidly progressed through the ranks. The vintage Bentley he drove as a student didn't go unnoticed, either.

Naturals

Are there 'naturals'? Are there doctors and nurses born for medical practice? One might regard those born with all the prerequisite talents as 'naturals', but some of them will decide that medicine is not for them. Those who decide to practise medicine will still need preparation and practice.

Besides the gift, you need the drive.
Neil Sedaka.

Those with a natural talent rarely need conscious calculation to do their job. They are quietly confident of their know-how. I have little doubt that innate talent exists, although for those who possess it, the first step is to become aware of it. The next step is to find the drive to use it effectively.

NBW: Nasty Bits of Work

It's not enough for me to win. My friends must lose.
                                         Gore Vidal.

My son Nicholas, a commercial airline pilot with Easy Jet, recently had a skin naevus inspected by a dermatologist. Flying exposes pilots to more UV light than usual and a high risk of skin cancer. Once the cosmetic surgeon learned for whom he worked, he asked: 'I suppose that means you failed to become an RAF pilot?' Nicholas replied: 'That's an interesting question. I rejected the idea of joining the RAF because I wouldn't have wanted to bomb innocent people!' (Nicholas is a typical JGG, and the cosmetic surgeon a typical NBW.)

One must approach all rude and challenging people with care. Some of their gratification will come from putting people down. Like angry dogs, they can attack (verbally) without warning. Few have more bite than bark, but one can't assume it. Frustration and hormonal changes can add to their grumpiness. Some are not getting what they want from life, but nothing should excuse their unpleasant behaviour. There can be a bipolar element to their nature: nasty or affable, depending on their mood swings and motives. Unless we choose more affable and predictable characters to befriend, the prospect of *schadenfreude* is likely.

Nice

To meet genuinely nice people is a wonderful thing. Beware, though, being nice is sometimes a manipulative gambit.

NPC

In the computer gaming world, they recognise Non-Playable Characters, or NPCs. Some doctors and nurses, when pressed, will do their best not to get involved. For this reason, GPs can find it difficult to get deserving and urgent medical cases into hospital. Those answering their call can be NPCs and very unhelpful; some will practice their excuses for not accepting patients. In response, some UK GPs will tell their patients to go to A&E, and to bypass the admissions system.

Does every hospital ward have one? A person who floats around with a clipboard, hoping not to get involved.(See: Shifting Dullness)

Obsessives and Nit-Pickers

Whoever thinks a faultless piece to see.
Thinks what ne'er was, nor is, nor e'er shall be.

Alexander Pope. *An Essay on Criticism* (1711). Part 2: 253-254.

Q. Can you spot a truly obsessional person?
A. Of course. They eat alphabet spaghetti in alphabetical order!

Because medicine is partly driven by medico-legal considerations these days, nit-pickers have come into their own. Obsession is a double-edged sword. It can foster meticulous work or distract attention from the job in hand. Some doctors and nurses may be so keen to get every 'i' dotted, and every 't' crossed, they may not notice a patient deteriorating. Their drive is to complete the task in hand, regardless of relevance. They can often do only one thing at a time. When there is a need for urgent clinical action, their inability to finish what they are doing could put lives at risk.

I have often instructed colleagues to end their telephone call, or stop whatever they were doing (chatting, or looking at a mobile phone screen), in order to focus on the clinical action. The ability to prioritise clinical situations, and drop everything when necessary, is an essential characteristic for emergency doctors, nurses and paramedics. Some obsessive characters will fail the challenge.

Consider what happened on the flight deck of United Flight 173, when flying from New York to Portland, Oregon, on the 28th December 1978. The two pilots flying the DC8 had thousands of hours of flying experience between them.

As they approached Oregon, a false warning light appeared, suggesting failed landing gear deployment. Actually, a damaged sensor light misled the pilots. The flight crew held the airplane in a holding pattern while they discussed the problem. By the time they decided on their readiness to

land, with the airport in sight and emergency vehicles stand-
ing by, 70 minutes had passed - 5 minutes longer than they
had fuel for. Their engines flamed out one by one, and they
crash-landed, ploughing through several houses. They skid-
ded to a halt after 500 yards. Most of the passengers lived.
There was no fire because they had burned every drop of fuel.
Their obsessive checking of lists and options had drawn their
attention away from one crucial flight instrument – the fuel
gauge!

Exactitude is important in many disciplines, but can be misplaced. There was, for instance, no point in taking an inventory of deck-chairs on the Titanic as she was sinking. It did perhaps help to avert anxiety. Obsessional people make good proof-readers, and safety checkers, but can be so concerned with the detail, they miss the wider picture.

Fear of failure drives many academic achievers; they fear of missing an important detail. Many are obsessional about detail. Few patients will warm to a surgeon who feels it necessary to list all 14 known complications of the operation they are about to perform (regardless of the in-dividual probabilities). This behaviour might comply with good medical practice, but it can diminish patient trust and confidence. For some patients, this will represent a failure to use the art of medicine.

Old Bailey Types

Every conversation is adversarial. They will call for doc-umentary evidence, the definition of any terms used, and justification for everything said. Relating to them can be hard work.

Old Vic Types

Every inter-reaction with them is a drama. Beware of taking a role in their play.

OOSOOM: *Out Of Sight, Out Of Mind*.

When a doctor or nurse asks their colleague for help, it could be the last they see of them. Why would that be? Are they selfish, or just too busy? Either way, they are unreliable and best avoided. Sorry to repeat it, but when trying to understand people, the direction their feet take is often more revealing than their words.

OVIBOI: OVerly Impressed By his /her Own Importance.

Such people are self-possessed, conceited and vain. There is only one important seat at any table – theirs. Their needs must take priority. Collect lots of evidence prior to any discussion with them and use it to counter their self-centred views. This will not endear them to you, and with luck, it will encourage them to avoid you.

Try this as a zoning-out exercise that no Russian speaker will appreciate. They much dislike their language being adulterated. OVIBOI is not a Russian word, but it sounds like one. If it were not an English acronym, it would rhyme with Bolshoi (masculine for 'Big' in Russian, like the famous Moscow theatre). It is linguistic nonsense to suggest that a doctor could be a Bolshoi OVIBOI (if male). The female equivalent (also nonsense) would be a Bolshaya OVIBAYA. A few British people might find this suggestion faintly amusing; no Russian will. Humour is a culturally sensitive issue.

OWT: One **W**ay **T**raffic.

Although doctors and nurses give of themselves, and try to help others when possible, others will not always reciprocate with the same generosity of spirit. If you find this upsetting, learn to select your associates more carefully.

Pedantic Pedagogues

The original Greek derivation of pedagogue is from 'rules' (*agoge*), applied to 'children' (*paidia*), like the rules of conduct written by a schoolmaster for his pupils. Medically trained pedagogues are in plentiful supply. They are doggedly adherent to rules, regardless of the benefits or downsides. The trait will diminish their ability to make diagnoses, especially with 'difficult' cases. They should consider a job in administration.

Only pedants will enjoy this fact. The Greek phrase 'Oi Polloi' means 'the people' ('Oi', in Greek, means 'the'). If you say 'The Oi Polloi', you will be saying 'the, the people.' That's pedantic.

Persona Non Grata (PNG)

For the delivery of any message, there will always be one who is the most effective messenger. A child might completely ignore its mother when commanded not to twirl their hair or pick their nose. Their teacher at school will more likely be obeyed after delivering the same message (perhaps because the entire class might overhear). The fact is, some messengers are more effective than others.

It is important to consider who might be the best person to deliver a message to a patient. The most appropriate person might be a relative, a colleague or a friend. In the relationship between messenger and patient, status, age group, culture, and gender are all relevant factors. If the object is to convey understanding and appreciation, the best person for the job might not be a doctor or nurse.

Ignaz Philipp Semmelweis was the Hungarian gynaecologist who discovered that fever after childbirth occurred only after patients were examined by doctors who had just returned from mortuary dissection. Washing their hands prevented it, although not then the accepted practice. He presented his data to colleagues in a form that they found unintelligible; he thus failed to convince them of his observations. In addition, his background was not prestigious enough to command their respect. His important discovery therefore remained unacknowledged.

Florence Nightingale nearly suffered a similar fate, but she presented her Crimean medical data in a novel, understandable format. She invented the first pie-chart to do so. That she was an aristocrat with many vital political and social connections must also have helped her case.

Phraseologists

Some doctors excel at expressing themselves in politically correct, one-upmanship phrases that will win them credit with colleagues. Doctors with an extensive stock of 'in vogue' phrases are more likely to be thought competent. Those who use phrases such as 'time-critical', 'fit-for-purpose', 'statistical significance', 'evidence-based', 'quality of life issue', or who use clinical trial acronyms, will make an impression. Those who use these shorthand, headline phrases do not always understand them fully. Some use them as rhetorical devices to convince others of their competence.

When left undefined, the use of an obscure acronym for a research trial might imply that everyone present knows all about the research. Latin phrases will similarly impress. Few will dare ask for a translation. Few wish to display their ignorance.

PIMP: Power Is My Purpose

Plenty of doctors seek power. Committees, steering groups, and political organisations like the British Medical Association, Royal Society of Medicine, and the Royal Colleges attract them. Perhaps they should consider a full-time political career, and aim to become Minister for Health. That would be a first. Nobody has yet seen the merit of appointing a Minister of health with a medical or nursing qualification and the appropriate clinical experience.

PITA: Pain In The Arse

Some are doctors, a few are nurses. It would be a pain in the arse to describe them further. They come in many annoying and tedious varieties. They commonly induce sly comments and the eye-rolling of bystanders.

Socrates gained a reputation for asking annoying but pertinent questions. He became known as the Gadfly of Athens.

PLASMA: A Person Lacking Any Sort of Medical Acumen.

PLOJ: A **P**erson **L**acking **O**bservable **J**udgement.

PLOP: A **P**erson **L**acking any **O**bservable **P**ersonality.

Politicians

Some doctors get involved in both local and nationwide politics. They might help more patients through political change than by practising medicine. They will quickly pass you by as they climb the ladder to their intended public office.

Many bureaucrats believe the path to medical utopia must be paved with regulation manuals. I would prefer to see it laid with mosaics depicting nurses and doctors throughout the ages; those freely using their clinical judgement and experience to help patients.

The doctor-patient relationship may not provide power enough for politically minded nurses and doctors. They might, however, come to represent us all in the halls of power. Their political mission might sometimes conflict their personal medical mission.

Preppies

Those who prepare well and practice often.

Pretty People and Charisma

Only a few precious beings have charisma, undoubted beauty, and star quality. Through no fault of their own, they easily incite staring and jaw-dropping interest in others. A queue of obsequious, lip-licking, eyelash fluttering, 'come and take me whenever you want' people, may trail behind them hoping for one small crumb of recognition.

Actress Mae West prescribed how to get noticed: tell the beautiful they are smart, and smart they are beautiful.

Leslie Phillips played the ultimate smooth operator while playing the character Dr. Gaston Grymsdyke. No actor has ever said 'Hello', with more licentious lasciviousness. (See films like 'Doctor in Clover', Rank Organisation, 1966).

Quants

For stock market analysis, quants do the calculations and weigh the risks of trading deals. In medicine, the same types also exist. Many are what used to be called 'back-room boys.' Valuable colleagues, but not always best placed at a patient's bedside.

RA: Risk Averse, and Not Risk Averse (NRA)

A practicable sense of risk is not possible without considerable clinical experience. Gamblers have an advantage. Those who regularly play roulette know the exact odds of winning or losing. With one zero slot, and 36 other numbers on a roulette wheel (some have a zero and a double zero), the chance of the ball dropping into any one slot is 37:1. If you play with these odds long enough, you will get a feel for the likelihood of winning. Those who despise games of chance will be at a disadvantage. They will find it difficult to put the odds of winning or losing into numerical perspective.

Most people prefer predictability to unpredictability. Many, in fact, have a neurotic desire for predictability, and become anxious without it. They may find it difficult to take risks, even though everything done in life carries a risk. Doctors soon become accustomed to the fact that medical practise is inherently risky, whether performing emergency surgery, or reporting MRI scans. The risk of error and patient suffering is ever present.

For interventional doctors (surgeons and cardiologists), risk aversion can inhibit action; interventional cardiology is not for the circumspect. Procrastination can prove dangerous. There is some advantage for patients who have a risk averse surgeon. They will operate only when they are 100% sure of their success rate. In very dire surgical situations, however, patients can be better off with a surgeon who will try his best, even when the risks are high. In the last-chance saloon, there is nothing to lose and everything to gain.

I once knew a prestigious, older chest surgeon, who would only operate on very low-risk patients. His patients were all fit and had the best indications for surgery. He had a 100% operative success rate, but operated on very few patients. Be careful how you interpret the reputation of physicians and surgeons. Their criteria for selecting patients and their position on the risk-aversion scale are important when choosing to refer to them.

Only non-risk averse doctors will dispense with caution and get on with the job. Although they will save lives, many will think them reckless and cavalier if things go wrong. Around them will be doctors fearful, and frozen to the spot, unable to contemplate any risk at all. They might not see the danger of inactivity. For the most effective doctors, risk-aversion is a variable; one that is altered case by case.

Important factors influence patient risk evaluation: the patient's general fitness (often related to length of illness), their clinical viability (some patients are tough, while others are frail), and likely complications (given specific predispositions like clotting or infection). To assess the risk, doctors need to combine these considerations with the technical difficulty of the procedure and the skill of the operator.

I was working in Casualty in 1967, when a road traffic accident victim arrived. The patient was pale, sweaty, in pain, and semi-conscious. He slipped into unconsciousness as an Egyptian surgeon strode in and called for a scalpel, sterile gloves, i.v. drips in both arms, blood for immediate infusion, and an anaesthetist (me). He demanded an operating theatre to be prepared – straight away! With no time wasted on explanations, he made an upper abdominal incision, inserted a gloved hand into the abdomen, and compressed the patient's spleen. We then rushed several hundred metres to the nearest operating theatre, where he performed an emergency splenectomy. The patient survived.

The experience was inspiring. I knew then I wanted to be involved in this sort of action. I later did similar things in cardiac emergencies. It is an edifying privilege to rescue patients from the jaws of death.

A pathologist once called our cardiac team to attend the hospital autopsy room ASAP. What the pathologist showed us was a pacing wire, previously inserted by me during resuscitation. It had not entered a vein as intended, but the arch of the patient's aorta. I had advanced the catheter into the left ventricle (not the right ventricle as usual via a vein), with no internal haemorrhage at all. The patient paced successfully until his death from renal failure.

The patient had been blue-lighted with a police escort to our cardiac team at St. George's, Hyde Park Corner, London. Too few doctors then knew much about emergency cardiac pacing. The patient's heart had stopped, and he was on the floor of a ward, as I entered the scene. Chest compression was being performed, and must have squeezed his major artery (aorta) up towards his collar bone. I inserted a pacing electrode effortlessly, and he paced successfully within 20 seconds. No X-ray was available at the location to check the position of the pacing electrode. The dark blood that came back through the entry needle appeared to come from a vein. In retrospect, it must have been dark, de-oxygenated arterial blood.

A word of caution about risk taking. There is a thin line between correct NRA action and recklessness. I never once met a reckless surgeon who could not resist operating. Inertia is the more common problem in emergency situations, with some doctors and nurses frozen to the spot with a patient bleeding to death in front of them. I have classified these as 'BBC's', 'PLASMAs', 'SDs', 'USBs' and 'RAs.' Some doctors have no instinct for rapid assessment and action. They should give serious thought to treating acne as a specialty.

When any bureaucrat gets involved with medical risk assessment, challenge what they might know about it, without ever having faced the sort of situations illustrated above. Challenge their assumptions and their actual experience.

Reliable / Unreliable

Patients need reliable doctors; those who turn up on time and do what is necessary. Unreliable doctors and nurses are potentially dangerous.

The surgeon I appointed for one of my patients put off her abdominal operation for bowel obstruction. It was Friday, and he had plans for the weekend. The delay left this anxious patient worrying about her diagnosis, the surgery she faced and her fate. I replaced him with a surgeon who operated on her a few days later. She was so exhausted by then, her immune system failed to cope. She died of septicaemia post-operatively.

Romantics

Dr. Negativo: 'I hate medicine.'

Dr. Positiva: 'No, you don't. You love it. Loving it is what you hate!'

Instead of objectivity, some doctors prefer the romantic view of their past achievements and what they might achieve in the future. They may come to support romantic, patient oriented ideas, like 'one can be forever young' (if only they had the best cosmetic surgeon), or, 'every cloud has a silver lining' (after consulting the best doctor; taking the best advice, or submitting to the right operation). A few doctors are true romantics, cock-eyed optimists who could have been talented actors.

Romantically inclined doctors can encourage hope, and nobody ever died from that. Problems lie with false hope and false expectation. Doctors must discourage patients from having procedures that are unlikely to improve their situation. In terminal, dire, or inevitable situations, false hope can be hurtful. Only those who know their patients well enough should exaggerate hope. If it improves the patient's composure, it will sometimes improve their prognosis.

There is plenty of evidence to suggest that grief diminishes survival. This is not a new concept.

In 1630, the Company of Parish Clerks in London reported twenty who died of parental 'Grieffe', perhaps because of the death of their child. The death of young children and infants was then commonplace. Two thousand, three hundred and twenty-eight 'Chrisomes' (children less than one month old) and infants, died in that year. Plague killed 1091, while other causes of death were age (662), 'bloody flux' (438), childbirth (157), and stillbirth (423).

A romantic notion, rather than the plain unmitigated truth, will sometimes encourage patients to beat the odds, if only for a while. Using hope appropriately is not an art possessed by all doctors. The art of medicine might dictate that a bare-faced lie is expedient. If I thought a lie would benefit a patient in the short-term (when their prognosis was poor), or in the long-term (if their prognosis was unknown), I never hesitated. Deception is now discouraged as unethical, and poor practice. That will suit all those doctors and administrators with a detached view of medical practice, and those who want anonymity. They will usually have little talent for the art of medicine.

I well remember talking to one of my best friends, Tony Smith, about what we would do together once he recovered his strength and left the hospice. Even though his prognosis from widespread melanoma was bleak, we made plans. Although we both tacitly accepted that our ideas were romantic, it helped us both cope with the inevitable. I was not his doctor. I had a more important role to play as his best friend.

Tony and I met at school when we were 11-years-old. We sat together in class. On a school holiday when we were both 13-years-old, we found ourselves abandoned late one night in Riccione, Italy. A taxi driver said he could take us no further than the edge of town. We had to walk the rest of the way to the Albergo Alba D'Oro, in Rimini. We started our 12Km. walk in darkness, at 11.30pm. and arrived back around 1.30am. Tony was forever positive, a cheerful boy, never easily disheartened. This was well before the invention of mobile telephones, so we couldn't let our teachers know where we were. They must have been frantic with worry.

Tony's enthusiasm for life, and that walk in particular, stays with me. What a gift to have a wise and joyful companion for life's journey. It naturally fell to me to encourage him while he was taking his last steps. I still treasure our friendship, and the mutual trust and faith we found in one another. I am happy to have helped his composure in his last days, as we reminisced about our happy school-days and made future plans. Encouraging him in a light-hearted way brought him some peace. Our long companionship served us well. Memories of his wise council stay with me and still guide my decisions today. (Alaya Ha-Shalom).

Ruthless

Some doctors ruthlessly pursue their career by cultivating the favour of senior colleagues, and bypassing or denigrating those of little use to them. Other doctors should avoid them completely; they will leave a trail of dejected souls in their wake.

Scammers

In private medicine, some doctors have one over-riding aim: to make money. Some will escape the tight bureaucratic control of corporations like the NHS, in order to achieve it. Some will indulge in illegal scams or practises, contrary to the GMC's *Good Medical Practice* guide, and not always in any patient's interest.

One innocent scam I came across involved referrals to a private hospital for cardiac CT scans. I had made hundreds of such referrals to private hospitals, but I had never referred a patient to one particular private hospital. It surprised me to learn that each patient referred had to be seen by their 'in-house' cardiologist. From this, he generated a fee. There is nothing wrong with suggesting a second opinion, but this unnecessary intervention seemed a scam to both me and my patient.

Other quasi-scams have been around for decades. One involves the cross-referral in the private sector to professional friends and colleagues. The effect is for them to get extra income, and for the patient referrer to be granted support in the future. Second opinions, and opinions from those in different specialties, can be highly desirable, but sometimes unnecessary. There can be a minor scam element to the practice, since the patient will have to pay a lot more in extra fees.

Unnecessary (or difficult to justify) follow-up consultations is another quasi-scam some private patients complain about, especially when each follow-up consultation is costly. This is a common, but inevitably limited practice. It is short-sighted because it will disincline patients to seek follow-up assessments, and could diminish a doctor's future long-term potential. That will not concern most private (also NHS based) consultants because few will see the same patient more than once.

Private medical insurers have long known that some private practices add unnecessary extra costs to insured patient accounts. Other payors, like oil-rich foreign embassies, care little about any such extras. For decades, they have paid unquestioningly for scarcely justifiable investigations, and much longer stays in London private hospitals than necessary (daily visits by doctors also add a lot to their account). Because these practices are only loosely justifiable, they are best referred to as quasi-scams.

Scary Guys

Jack Nicholson, when acting, was often told to 'lose the scary look.'

A few doctors have a 'mad look' in their eyes. Fixed, starring eyes, and exposed conjunctivae are a universal, non-verbal sign of danger. If they are stern and abrupt as well, few will want to approach them. A kindly pussy cat mentality can hide behind a scary face, but few will be brave enough to test it. Patients should have feared Dr. Harold Shipman, but they didn't. I believe he was kind and affable, and not scary at all. He apparently had a supportive and unassuming manner which endeared him to many patients. What other doctors thought of him, I do not know.

Scholar

These are intellectual doctors, interested in medical science and scholarship but little else. They deserve respect. Although, often high-minded, the trait does not exclude a talent for executive functioning, compassion and the art of medicine.

The Selfless Few

Those who can deal selflessly with the baseness of humanity are saints. Typically, they are shy and self-effacing and not at all interested in seeking recognition. In common with those worthy of the Victoria Cross, they feature modesty and no taste for self-promotion. Such people are rare, but a few exist in the medical profession; all healthcare workers are potential candidates. Despite my cynicism about some doctors, the possession of these traits is something for the medical profession to be proud of.

Two doctors won the Victoria Cross twice: Lt. Col. Surgeon Arthur Martin-Leake, and Captain Noel Chavasse.

Captain Charles Upham, a New Zealand soldier, also won it twice but was not a doctor.

Elizabeth W. Harris (1834 – 1917) was the only woman (nurse) to receive (a replica of) the Victoria Cross (1869). Queen Victoria gave special permission for this. It was for her bravery during a cholera outbreak in India. She remains the only woman to be awarded a VC of any description. Only since 1921 have women been eligible to receive a VC. Not one has been won since.

Serious All The Time (SATT)

These doctors and nurses are never light-hearted, and working with them can be hard work. Some appear to be weighed down by the gravity of their status and knowledge. Many share aspects of Asperger's. See also: 'PITA.'

SD: Shifting Dullness

This applies to those nurses and doctors who float around from one place to another, looking busy, but doing very little. They usually move in the shadows (many holding a clip-board), hoping to avoid work, decision making, or any sort of meaningful involvement. As avoidance behaviour, they may hope not to have their incompetence discovered. Many are simply lazy. It Paradoxically, some become well thought of. This is because they have employed the simplest of strategies - minimal offensiveness.

Slobs

Doctors and nurses are not immune to smelling offensive ('body odour'). This will offend both patients and most other staff. It will fall to someone brave enough to point it out to them. They might suggest that soap is cheap, or that regular washing is a usual necessity. It is common in nerds and those with a solitary nature. Never overlook the possibility of their deteriorating mental health or psychiatric illness; uncleanliness can result from failing to cope, depression, and psychosis.

If you are unsure of what a slob might be, go to YouTube, and search for Harry Enfield's *The Slobs*, Wayne and Waynetta. I have met only one or two doctors who emulated them: they failed to wash consistently, only rarely changed their clothes, comb their hair or tidy their rooms. Some will ignore piles of unwashed dishes, and in years gone by, never emptied their ashtrays. In the 1960s, many doctors and nurses smoked; it helped them cope with the stress of medical work (one of the few benefits of smoking), while ignoring lung cancer risk (a concept then in its infancy).

Because behaviour provides an accurate guide to the true nature of a person, the disinterest of slobs in cleanliness says a lot about them and their attention to detail. Is there a connection between a tidy home and a tidy mind? The Victorians thought so. They thought 'cleanliness next to Godliness.' Obviously eccentric, absent-minded intellectuals, with their minds on higher things can overlook self-care. Others are just lazy.

During World War 2, Alan Turing, while making ground-breaking advances in computer technology and cipher analysis (requiring the ultimate sort of tidy mind), would often arrive for work at Bletchley Park wearing pyjamas. Unkempt, he may have been, but a genius none-the-less.

Someone I trust most as an expert on human behaviour (C.D.) once told me:

'Employ no-one who comes for an interview wearing dirty shoes. If they don't take care of their shoes, they won't take care of their duties.'

Smart

Shrewd people always do their reconnaissance. They come to know their true situation from every angle, and then correctly position themselves to take advantage. The medical profession is replete with shrewd guys, all trying to feather their nests (professionally and financially). This makes recognition of this trait an important one for the naïve, tender-hearted, weak-willed, trusting, and inexperienced. It is especially important for nerds whose minds are elsewhere.

In Confucianism, smartness alone is not enough; it must combine with 'Ren 口', to form wisdom. Crudely translated, 'Ren' is the virtue of combining understanding with humanity.

Smoothies

Oleaginous, suave and self-assured, they often speak in mellifluous tones, and ooze composure and confidence. They are mostly harmless.

In both films 'Doctor in Clover' (1966. Rank Organisation), and 'Doctor in Love' (1960. Rank Organisation), actor Leslie Phillips plays the archetypal smoothie.

Spanophilia(c).

A term used by Richard Asher *(Talking Sense.* 1972. Pitman). The word is used to describe an undue interest in obscure medical conditions. Some doctors will find any excuse to introduce their much loved diagnostic hobby horse into every discussion (it thus appears to be an obsession). This can be harmless as a hobby or a research interest. It otherwise risks detracting from a balanced view of a patient's clinical picture. Found in researchers, spanophilia can motivate discovery.

One of my 'A' level biology teachers, Dr. W.B. Broughton, was a renowned UK grasshopper specialist. He gave his name to one: Chorthippus broughtensis, one of three English grasshoppers, then named. Dr. Broughton taught me between 1959-61, and because he was searching for a fourth grasshopper, had all his pupils, including me, scouring Epping Forest. We failed to find an undiscovered one. He was a memorable, inspiring teacher.

Star-Struck

Revering fame is not a passing weakness. For many, it fills their need for worship and reverence. I have seen patients fall stage-struck and starry-eyed at the feet of celebrity, although not all are sycophants. A chance meeting with someone famous might be their only chance of glory, if only reflected glory. Although a feeble source of self-esteem, it will enliven their story-telling. As a sign of their devotion, some will perform any task requested by their idol. They will happily demean themselves for one small scrap of recognition, and one faint promise of good-will.

Stern

According to Mark Forsyth (*The Elements of Eloquence*, p4, 2013, Icon Books) 'Stern people dislike rhetoric, and unfortunately, it is stern people who are in charge: solemn fools who believe that truth is more important than beauty.'

Some stern academics get weighed down by the gravity of their status and knowledge.

The incompetence of some stern people will lie hidden. Many fear them and lack the courage to challenge them. Few naturally stern characters have a hidden sense of humour. Some might explain that it was only after suffering too many fools that they adopted a stern outlook.Some then find it expedient to presume that everyone is stupid until proven otherwise. Adopting a stern approach is an excellent way to cut short any inane conversation.

The perfect image of a stern doctor is *Doc Martin* (played by Martin Clunes in the UK, TV series (2004-2009), the creation of Dominic Minghella. In reality, Martin is not at all stern; he is just a great actor.

Stern characters often display other unpleasant traits: rudeness, arrogance and incompetence.

Stressed Doctors

'. . . *those restless thoughts which corrode the sweets of life.*'

Izaak Walton.
The Compleat Angler (1653).

The work of doctors and nurses can bring them enough stress to induce panic attacks, anxiety, depression, and an inability to cope. They may have had to work long hours, with sleep deprivation, and had to suffer trouble at home, problems with their finances, and illness in their family. This may have caused them to get tired and exhausted and to look haggard. The face of US President Richard Nixon after Watergate, and that of Tony Blair after Chilcot, (facing the threat of legal action against his actions 13-years before), once provided graphic examples.

After long periods of stress, some get depressed. Others make promises they cannot keep, lose their sense of humour, and their sense of timing and reliability. They may fail to 'get themselves together'. To make matters worse, they make more mistakes than usual. They will need to sleep and get help with what has caused their demise. Many take to alcohol, and a few to drugs; neither help in the long-term. They are prone to 'Knight's Move' decision making and action. These are ill-researched, life-changing moves, taken to relieve the pressure and urgency they find unbearable. Some will suddenly re-sign their job, move house, join the Foreign Legion or go off to help in a leper colony with very little fore-thought. They can be strangely resistant to accept the help they need most. They may see accepting help as an admission of weakness and a loss of face. When recognised, we should advise them, support them and help them whenever possible.

Structured and Unstructured Thinkers

There are those who always need a plan to follow. Without one, they can lose their composure and become anxious and insecure. They don't mind being in a maze, as long as they have a map to go with it. What they abhor is a lack of guidance. Some feel secure only when they are following rules.

Structured thinkers need to work in a strictly defined environment, with accepted rules and regulations to follow. They will get anxious if called upon to use their nous, to think for themselves, or to make judgements and decisions based on insufficient information.

In order to galvanise their people together, both Jewish and Islamic religions, have long provided compendia of rules and practices for every occasion (for Jews, The Shulchan

Aruch; Sharia for Moslems). The most devout follow them to the letter.

There are others with no wish to be restricted by rules and regulations; they prefer the freedom to think, to be creative and to invent new things. They enjoy lateral thinking and solving problems, and will enjoy engaging with the mysterious and the unknown. In flying terms, they can 'fly by the seat of their pants', and like the first pilots, will find out what counts as they go along. They know the value of experience and never lose sight of it when thinking. As adaptable, resourceful, and creative creatures, they see few limits to their problem solving.

Stüm(mer) (*Yiddish. Pronounced: 'shtummer.' Derived from 'mute' in German.*)

A taciturn person, with whom conversation is hard work. They are mostly silent, non-responsive types who cannot, or will not, express their feelings. Some are good listeners. Some are simply shy initially, and will 'open up' later. They become activated when discussing their favourite topics. Some are autistic. I have always found it strange that stümmers are often credited with superior knowledge.

There can be a sinister side to a patient remaining mute. A person being dominated may be afraid to speak, especially in the presence of their dominator / dominatrix. The history they give may be filtered. Safeguarding issues then arise. The central questions are whether anyone else is in control, and whether that control needs to be challenged. What are the motives, and who is to gain? Never jump to

conclusions: those patients with retarded development
or senile dementia need well-intentioned guidance.

'SS': Supercilious and Sanctimonious

These are common enough traits found in doctors,
but not so much in nurses. These attitudes may be
'in-born', but for political reasons, not always on display. They are much more likely to be observed while
doctors are dealing with their patients than with their
colleagues. Some share features with OVIBOI types.
There is a cultural element to these traits, associated
with wealth, education and security.

Swimmers and Sinkers

After being thrown into deep clinical water, the coping ability of an inexperienced doctor or nurse will soon
be clear.

My first surgical registrar was a visiting Australian
surgeon, Colin Davis ('Col'). He told me on my first day
of work: 'Dave, I'm a cutter. I know very little about
medical matters. If it's a medical case, it's all down to
you. If it's surgical, call me.'

'Col', handed me the opportunity to find out what I
was capable of; a chance very few will ever get these days
in the UK, regulations and paternalistic attitudes being as
they are. Having found myself in deep water not knowing

whether I could swim, I soon swam away and never looked back.

I would argue that if medical schools wanted to choose medical students who will cope well with medical practice, they should check their coping ability by exposing them to cases in A&E, before accepting them as medical students. When thrown into fast-running, deep water, only the lucky and the strongest swimmers will survive. They can then save the lives of others.

I know, all this sounds inegalitarian and over the top, but reflect on the fact that the practice of medicine IS a serious matter, and IS often dangerous, and a degree of courage is necessary to handle it well. Lives are at stake, and this is no place for the weak-minded or weak-hearted. That's OK, there are thousands of places in the medical world where shuffling bits of paper is the primary function and much less risky.

Team Players

Like the rest of humanity, we can divide doctors and nurses into loners (squash players, golfers, and chess players), and team players (rugby, and football players). Both types have made notable contributions to science, medicine, and medical science.

Sporting doctors who are team players will thrive in multidisciplinary units. When I worked there, the pacing unit at St. George's, Hyde Park Corner, was one such place; although my only claim to team playing was having rowed in an eight for my school and medical college.

Although a loner, I much enjoyed working in a small, tightly integrated team of capable professionals. Top-rate collaborators make development work easy.

Unfortunately, NHS bureaucrats with little or no clinical wisdom once considered disbanding one such crack clinical team. In 2016, they tried to close the Paediatric Cardiology Unit at the Royal Brompton Hospital. They doubtless thought it uneconomic. It called into question whether they understood anything of how doctors, nurses, and patients work best together. In December 2017, perhaps having learned something of how well-developed teamwork counts, they reversed their decision.

Giving authority to bureaucrats with insufficient medical knowledge, no experience, and even less ability is surely an insult to stupidity.

How much more untutored intervention do UK doctors and nurses need to suffer from bureaucrats? Read my book '*The NHS. Our Sick Sacred Cow*' to read what I think, and what I think should be done about it.

Thin Skinned. Thick Skinned.

Those doctors and nurses impervious to criticism, we call thick-skinned. They have either learned from experience how to counter criticism, or have enough confidence to ignore it.

Ex-US President Donald Trump is reported to have 'A fat ego in a thin skin.' (PennLive, March 2017: Bob Quarteroni).Trump says of himself, 'I have very strong, very thick skin.'

When Trump was president, was he easily hurt by criticism, and did he react in resentful ways? With his experience of running businesses, I think it just as likely that administrators who knew much less about the real world of business than him, caused him endless frustration.

Types A & B

Although 'time urgency' (Type A behaviour) is an important behavioural characteristic of doctors, it is perhaps more important to recognise it in patients. I have deferred describing these traits until the next chapter.

USBN: USeless But Nice.

A few doctors and nurses seem not to know much and are inept at performing practical procedures. They find venesection, lumbar puncture, and establishing i.v. infusions too challenging.

I once worked with a charming, much older junior doctor, who would co-opt his colleagues to help him with every practical procedure. His ambition was to become a child psychiatrist. He saw no point in practising procedures he found difficult, that were unpleasant for patients, and were

irrelevant to his future. He was wealthy, and to salve his con-
science, often had Fortnum and Mason's hampers delivered
to our ward. We forgave his ineptitude.

Uptight and Buttoned-up

Many people are unrevealing by nature and keep their
cards close to their chest. Doctors and nurses are no exception. They will want to know everything about you, but
tell you nothing about themselves. Those with an autistic
trait are different; they may have little or interest in others
and may feel no need to reveal anything about themselves.
Some doctors are shy, others are hoping to gain control.
All of them present a communication problem.

Visionaries

Leonardo da Vinci and H.G. Wells were visionaries. I
was lucky to have encountered a few visionary doctors
myself (Dr. Aubrey Leatham, Dr. Peter Nixon, Dr. Alan
Gardner, Dr. Paul Kligfield, Dr. Pim de Feijter, Dr. David
Baxter, and Dr. Mike Hodges). All cultivated the future,
while working in the present. All were determined to make
their vision come to pass. Visionaries rarely benefit from
consulting with those grounded in the past, or those with
no vision of the future. If you have the courage for it, tag
along with one for an exciting ride.

Wimps

Yes, there are doctors and nurses who dislike the sight of blood, and who will run in the opposite direction when emergencies occur. They can feel ill, hyperventilate, and collapse at the sight of someone sick or injured. They will soon reveal themselves once they start work. If they don't consider a career in management or psychology, they could spend time as a patient themselves.

Wise Sage

We will all need wise advice sometime. We all get stuck while trying to make a diagnosis, or with a practical procedure, and need help. As doctors and nurses progress, it will be important for them to identify those who can be of most help, like those adept at practical procedures. Go to them and ask for help. There is no need to feel inferior or inadequate. By asking a wise, capable person, you help three people: the patient (who will suffer less trauma); you (who will have gained knowledge), and the one you asked (who will gain self-esteem).

CHAPTER TWO

PATIENT CARICATURES

Interested observers will often notice behavioural differences between people, especially when their age,
gender, culture and social class differs (social class is
still identifiable in the UK, using family background
and educational attainment). Those biased to accept
the political concept of equality might not be prepared
to recognise the wide spectrum of human behavioural
differences that exists between individuals. Will they
put undue emphasis on the fact that we all have more in
common than we have differences? Doctors and nurses
cannot afford this bias. We must first regard each patient as an incomparably different, unique individual.

One cannot deny biology and the behavioural differences between people. Political correctness attempts to
suppress this, even when subjected to a stronger force.
That force is evolution, selecting those fittest to survive
healthily and longest, based on our differences. Genetic
science and the practice of medicine are both attempting

to overcome evolution when they help those unfit for survival, to lead a normal life.

An equivalent holds true for zoo keepers. They need to generalise and recognise how each animal behaves differently (even those of the same species), in order to avoid being bitten, stung, or eaten alive. To remain safe, they must adopt some experienced-based generalisations, while admitting the many exceptions that must occur. Doctors need to adopt the same principles if they are to recognise different patient types and know how best to deal with each of them.

When thinking about human behaviour, we all have personal biases. For instance, those who only read broadsheet newspapers, watch BBC 2 and BBC 4 TV, and listen to Classic FM and BBC Radio 4, are likely to see others though a prism of UK middle-class values. Our social biases affect how compatible we feel meeting with those from socio-economic groups and cultures other than our own.

We can distinguish differences between individual social groups and cultures by using our impressions, or by referring to population surveys and statistical analyses for guidance. How reliable will be our impression of native behaviour when visiting a foreign country for the first time? Because our brains have none of the restraints of computer processing, we can freely form associations, impressions and judgements, although for evolutionary reasons we must first assess any danger. This type of functioning is more useful for survival than calculation. Humans can discriminate several directions at once, with our biases swaying us towards overrating risk or maximising hope. These may not be the most reliable of predictive cognitive functions, but they have sustained the survival of *homo sapiens* for millions of years.

Generalisations can provide us with preliminary fore-warnings. Experience will then suggest whether we should accept or reject them. Not all tigers will eat us as we enter their cage, but it is sensible to assume they will. A double-blind trial might confirm this presumption about tigers, but who would waste their time and money undertaking it? (The answer is, of course, a government department, or a tax funded corporation like the NHS). Perhaps one should value common sense more and continue to presume that all tigers are dangerous.

The image, or 'face' that a patient presents, is the product of many influences: their rearing, their age, gender, culture, biases and personality; their socio-economic circumstances, intelligence, emotional intelligence, fears, neurotic traits and education, to mention but a few factors. Each of us holds only one genomic hand of cards with which to play the game of life. For the moment, we choose not to swap, substitute, or delete our genetic 'cards', although that possibility is not far off.

In all card games, there is a distinct advantage to knowing the cards held by the opponents. Life circumstances might modify gene expression (epigenetics is now a popular concept), but no environmental circumstance known will cause a turkey grow wings, and then soar into the sky like an eagle. We know, however, that radiation can cause cell mutation and cancer, but do not yet know whether the stresses of life will influence atherosclerosis and hypertension enough to cause heart attacks and strokes. The study of epigenetics is a work in progress.

The art of medicine requires a doctor to identify each patient as an individual. Individuals will soon be identifiable using their genetic profile, but to bring the maximum advantages of scientific medicine to individuals, given their circumstances, will still require doctors and nurses to practise the art of medicine.

In what follows, I have described all the patient types I have dealt with, and how relevant they have been to the doctor-patient relationship. These details are important, if only to forewarn inexperienced doctors and nurses of the pitfalls.

A natural overlap is inevitable when describing either patients, doctors or nurses as characters. The perception will differ, depending on whether it is a doctor or a patient reading the descriptions.

Patient Characters

Advantage Takers

Who would park their car in a disabled space (just for their convenience) when they have no disabled person in the car? Who will jump queues and show no regard for the patience of others?

Advantage takers are everywhere, and a few of them will be patients. They try their luck wherever they go. They will try to persuade medical practice receptionists that their problems are more urgent than they really are, just to jump the queue. See also Users.

ALAC: Acts Like a Child

This type of patient will usually have had their consultation arranged by a friend, relative, or workmate.
Their adopted role is passive, which can present a problem with co-operation. They can be in denial, or not
agree with the medical problem their friend thinks they
have. Paradoxically, they may become indignant if they
sense being treated like a child. Some will refuse to
accept advice; after all, they are under no obligation.
Those with more humility, might express some gratitude to the person who arranged their consultation.

*When I took John's full history, he denied any symptoms.
He did, however, have a strong family history of coronary
artery disease. His wife had sent him to get checked. He
was a 67-year-old golfer who played 18 holes of golf, 3
times every week. I knew the golf course. It was hilly. My
investigations included a carotid artery scan (this showed
heavily calcified atheromatous plaques, with a 95% occlusion on one side), and an ECG treadmill exercise test
which showed a significant problem.*

*We stopped his exercise test after only two minutes be-
cause he developed chest tightness and ominous ECG
changes associated with reduced coronary blood flow (ST
depression on his ECG). I questioned him further: 'I
thought you said you had no symptoms? How is it you can
play on a hilly golf course and not get chest tightness?' He
explained: 'It's easy. I use my buggy, and only get off it to
hit the ball. I then carry on. Without it I couldn't play
golf.'*

He had a small heart attack (cardiac infarction) two days later. His wife, supported by an A&E doctor, thought his diagnostic exercise test had caused his cardiac infarction (exercise testing is a sine qua non for cardiac ischaemia diagnosis in asymptomatic patients). He had an emergency CABG (coronary by-pass) one week later. He never returned to me as a patient; he and his wife blamed me for his heart attack.

He had ignored his failing health and had taken no personal responsibility for his condition. Given that he was behaving more like a child than an adult, he desperately needed guidance from a parent. Unfortunately for him, resurrecting his parents was not an available option.

Our duty must always be to the patient, never primarily to those who refer them. Doctors who respect professional etiquette above the welfare of their patients, may not agree. Some health professionals prefer to communicate only to the referring doctor, and not to the patient. It can lead to doctors not informing patients directly of the risks they face, and that lacks common sense.

Only the patient has any right to their clinical information. If they wish to give that information to family, friends or the company they work for, that is for them to decide.

ALBer: Arrogant **L**ittle **B**leeder.

This type of patient knows best, or thinks he does. They are demanding, and not disposed to listen.

The arrogant can be compliant, but only when it suits them. Presuming they know best, they may only comply when their opinion matches that of the doctor. These days, many patients use 'Doctor Google' as their source of medical information, and their compliance can depend on what they have read. Since many believe everything they read in newspapers, and what they find on the Internet, a lot of time can be wasted convincing them otherwise.

Arrogant beliefs pre-date the Internet by many millennia. Among the current ones are that antibiotics diminish immunity and prolong health problems (despite the many millions of lives they have saved); that special diets hold the secret to longevity, and that the avoidance of animal fat will prevent heart attacks. Some believe that gene-modified food and holding mobile phones will cause cancer. There are as many beliefs that concern the promotion of health as there are about the disease prevention and its cure.

Amateur Doctors

Experienced professionals in every field of work, have to suffer amateurs who think they know best. Just occasionally, one *will* know best. With an interest in medicine, science, the law, archaeology, or architecture, many amateurs have contributed novel theories and valuable observations. Others will jump to conclusions based on insufficient evidence and limited evaluation.

Jim had been an engineer and amateur brewer most of his life. He came to me with his irritable bowel syndrome (IBS), which had caused him stomach bloating from gas collection.
He asked if I would give him some anti-yeast medication and explained why. 'I am an amateur brewer, and I understand how gas is made when making beer. Sugar and yeast combine to produce carbon dioxide and alcohol, and I think this is happening in my bowel. If this is the case, I must have

a small amount of alcohol in my blood, so could you test my blood for it?

My reply was that I would research his blood alcohol theory.

Small amounts of blood are indeed detectable in the blood in those who have drunk no alcohol. It is now called the auto-brewery syndrome. When Jim suggested it to me over 30-years ago, I had never heard of it.

After Jim took some nystatin tablets used to treat yeast infections (his idea), he noticed no reduction in stomach bloating. He told me that his two sisters suffered similarly, and that the medication helped them.

Jim had come up with two new, scientifically plausible ideas. I had come across neither before.

Search engines are now a ready source of information for everyone; even those who would never have visited a library. Verified information, misinformation, and false information are all there on the world-wide-web, so I always encouraged patients to discuss what they had learned. The research they will do can be a good starting point, so why not provide them with some useful search terms. In depth discussion takes time - a valuable commodity, now rationed by the NHS.

Badly Behaved

In consulting rooms, some children will sit quietly while others talk. Others will roam around, opening cupboards, and removing anything that takes their fancy. Not all parents of such children admonish them; they will usually be the ones responsible for their behaviour. Most parents are euphemistic about their offspring. They will claim that they want to open cupboards because they are delightfully inquisitive research scientists in the making. There is another interpretation: they have yet to be domesticated. As with many other behavioural traits, family values and culture, shape us through their powerful influence.

When traveling, one will see differences in the behaviour of children from different cultural backgrounds. On internal Russian flights, you will rarely see a Russian child doing anything other than sitting quietly. Travel on a British, or a Mediterranean holiday flight, and you will be lucky to avoid occasional bedlam as unruly children run around unchecked. To add to this, their endearing, over-loudly chastising parents, will chase them down the aisles, half-heartedly apologising to onlookers as they go.

On airplanes, many travellers are now rich enough to reserve business class and first-class seats for their children. Some of them believe their children should be free to run amok whenever and wherever they wish. They have 'paid good money' to seat them in expensive seats, so why not? Why would others want to pay for a long-haul, first-class seat, and be exposed to such behaviour?

I was once on holiday in Corfu, having dinner at a family-owned taverna. The owner's mother was trying to coax her grandson to eat. To do this, she chased him around the tables with a teaspoon of food. All she had to do was hide the food and wait for him to get hungry. He would have come begging her for food. By allowing himself to be chased, this young boy was demonstrating the art of adult manipulation. He had learned the value of playing hard to get.

While all this was taking place, his grandfather was taking my order, and criticising my elementary Greek. I asked for a bottle of 'kokkino krasi' (literally 'red' wine). Not only did he tell me that the usual phrase was 'mavro krasi' (black wine), but where and when, I had learned my Greek. 'You have been watching 'Greek Language and People', Sunday nights, BBC 2. Too many mistakes', he said. He was a native Corfiot who lived in the UK during the winter months. I should have returned for more colloquial Greek lessons.

Children are not alone in displaying inappropriate behaviour.

Twenty-five-year-old Mark, a robust 20-stone kick-boxer, used to storm into my clinic without an appointment. With no preamble, he would ask my receptionist, 'Where's the doc? I need to see the Doc.' When he got to see 'the doc' (me), he would say, 'Doc, I feel like sh*t.' I would then ask him to give me a few clues. 'Is your throat sore, etc.' Because the level of communication between us was poor, I came to liken our meetings to veterinary consultations (with no pet owner present).

A few years later, Mark was found dead on a beach in Thailand. He had overdosed on a cocktail of drugs.

Can 'bad behaviour' signal a poor prognosis?

Bias Unaware

Every opinion is subject to personal bias. Cognitive biases were first publicised by Kahneman and Tversky in the 1970s. Their message was that everyone has biases that

influence their decision making and judgement processes, including those of patients, doctors and nurses.

Prevalent among student doctors and patients is the
'Halo' bias. The bias can weaken or strengthen their
belief in authority (teachers, for instance). The bias
promotes the assumption that those in authority know
best. Similarly, the public may view published writers,
media presenters, those with titles, and celebrities as
trusted sentient beings always to be believed. That is
the halo bias gone wrong. The same bias allows us to
view information on the Internet as definitive, true, and
not in need of challenge. Although unlikely, it could
cause a doctor to view patients who have gleaned a little
information from the Internet, as more knowledgeable
than they are.

A negative halo bias will lead us to under-rate others.
This is becoming more common for doctors. Patients
are becoming more questioning of what we know. Few
have any understanding of the knowledge required to
become a doctor or nurse.

Bereaved

Dealing with the bereaved is always challenging.
Those versed in the art of medicine will find it easier
than those gripped by the value of medical science. The
minimum requirement is for enough empathy and inter-personal responsiveness, to bring comfort to those
affected. There is an art to using the rhetoric of eulogy.

Blackmailers

Specifically, emotional blackmailers. This is an uncommon tactic used by some patients to get what they want from doctors. They will have used the same coercive force to get what they want from their friends and family. It is more likely to happen when patients 'get too close.' By 'too close', I mean sharing so much personal information with them, they come to regard their doctor or nurse as 'one of us'. This is more common in those cultures where 'who you know' is more important than 'what you know'.

BWMM: Butter **W**ouldn't **M**elt in their **M**outh.

They can be either a paragon of virtue, or a divisive criminal. Avoid being drawn into their vortex of influence.

Clever Guys

Well-educated, intelligent people will easily understand all the information you need to convey. They will want to discuss the data and the basis for your opinion. If they are not only clever, but wise, they will balance the information you give them with that from other sources. They will then decide what option best suits them.

A postgraduate physicist once consulted me. He thought we were all being controlled by high-energy, electromagnetic waves, broadcast by the government. His arguments were 'scientific' in nature, and his train of thought logical. The only problem was, his ideas were delusional. He was an untreated schizophrenic.

Some clever guys (including doctors) harbour strange, unsubstantiated beliefs, but are clever enough to present them as cogent. Although I have had a tendency to 'take

them on', I have learned with age to save my energy,
keep quiet, be graceful and move on.

Complainers (See Troublemakers)

In the West, we now accept our complaint-orient-
ed societies. This is the inevitable consequence of the
current political drive to achieve equal rights for all.
Many of the complaints now expressed by patients
in the NHS result from being mishandled, side-lined,
or ignored by those managing them. Being told that
the computer says 'NO', can induce behaviour that is
out-of-character. The inefficient handling of patients
under overload conditions is a common source of complaint. It never occurred in my practice. If frustration
or aggravation arose between my staff and a patient,
I stepped in immediately to arbitrate and sort it out.
Discord left too long can fester into anger and resentment. While decisive intervention can strengthen the
doctor-patient relationship, handling patients imper-
sonally can weaken it.

Every medical practice has a few patients who complain
a lot. Complaining is their modus operandi; a matter of
outlook, and even their mission in life. Classed as troublemakers wherever they go, they may enjoy the attention
it brings. When dealing with them, always ask for wit-
nesses to be present. A good receptionist will spot them
before they first attend as new patients. They are better
managed proactively than reactively. Gaining their respect
as *a person who listens*, and one who is fair and able to
resolve problems wisely, can allow for a bearable relationship. Beware of being too kind. Many complainers regard
kindness as a weakness; sensing kindness can cause them to
strengthen their attack. Although very time-consuming,

some complainers are worth listening to, especially if their criticisms are correct and constructive.

Complaints against doctors and nurses are fast-growing. If regulators are called to deal with them, it will place a doctor's career in jeopardy. Our regulators are there to listen, and must investigate every complaint made, charged as they are with protecting the public from evil, advantage-taking doctors and nurses with harmful practices. Because bureaucrats know so little about medicine, especially about how it functions at a personal level, they will assume that every complaint is true until proven otherwise. Devils lie in the detail, but with no knowledge of that detail, few know to ask the most pertinent and revealing questions. The personality and outlook of each complainant is one such detail; the true nature of the doctor and his practice is another. Since these questions will be beyond the remit of regulators, their judgements may be legally correct, but lack clinical perspective and appropriateness.

Patients need to be listened to. Sometimes, that is all they need. Bureaucrats entering the affray can alienate patients when direct intervention from the doctor involved would have settled the matter quickly. As all this fails, doctors and nurses must call their medical protection society at an early stage.

In private practice, every doctor needs a complaints policy. The first requirement is to listen. The second is to repeat the complaint back to the patient, confirming that you and she have both understand what is being alleged. Many minor complaints get resolved at this point. Whether or not resolved, one must write a contemporaneous report of each complaint in the patient's notes, with at least the account of one witness in writing. How the complaint was processed and resolved must be stated. Doctors and nurses have no option but to follow every element of corporate, medico-legal processing (rules and regulations devised by detached executives, in offices far, far away from reality), and to react in a predictable, stereotyped fashion. Doctors and nurses must avoid becoming victims of the well-oiled, corporate legal machine, currently employed to seek reasons for punishing doctors and nurses.

If the complaint escalates to involve lawyers, the medico-legal game will change completely. To the uninitiated, investigating allegations against doctors may appear to be moderate, respectful, clinically relevant, and considerate. Don't be fooled. It will be none of these.

Imagine being arrested for crimes and awaiting a trial. You could be about to get involved in an adversarial legal contest where the law, not medical matters, are the issue. Regulators then act as criminal investigators. Their mission is simple: to detect and punish any departure from the published rules (formed by the GMC's *Good Medical Practice*, NICE Guidelines, and the British National Formulary or BNF). They will not engage in clinical reasoning (they would appear incompetent if they did) and will dismiss the circumstantial and inter-personal details of your case as hearsay.

How regulators can expect to judge clinical situations fairly without relevant experience is an issue they never choose to address. Their concern is to judge compliance and to keep matters simple. The blame rests on the shoulders of the accused until proven otherwise. The law has given regulators the statutory right to enjoy the insolence of power. They need no respect for doctors or nurses whose vocation has been the relief of suffering, and the saving of lives. The legal complaint process is dis-passionate and can ignore balance, fairness, and what might be relevant clinical meta-data. The process of cross-questioning allows unfairness to be expressed, the exclusion of any clinical perspective, especially when it includes bullying and intimidation.

Our regulators need to be seen to keep the public safe. Some of them would like to bring back the stocks and humiliate doctors publicly. They have reasons for not going that far: it would be archaic and not win them favour with patients. Instead, they have adopted more modern, equally punishing methods: trial by tribunal (with usually only one GP present), and posting all their views of a doctor's misdemeanours on the internet for all to read. With their IT power, they can block any adverse comments about themselves. Doctors who try to retaliate, will not win without mounting a financial-ly crippling campaign. To retaliate effectively requires collective action, with help from internet savants (See also: Troublemakers).

Controllers

Those who desire to control others are ubiquitous. Avoid obsessional controllers working beyond their level of competence; some have a pathological fear of re-linquishing control. Being sure of their knowledge and ability, these patients may want to manage medical de-cisions personally. The process will fall apart when they attempt to interpret clinical data; in fact, the process can fall apart at any stage, leaving them perplexed.

What is it these patients (and some of our regulators) don't understand about the depth and breadth of a medical education, and the value of clinical experience? They may understand string theory better.

Although private patients can seek many opinions, they might only favour those who acknowledge their control. If they asked to remain conscious during a surgical operation, they could advise their surgeon where best to cut!

Cool Dudes

Look no further than Sean Connery's James Bond, or Winkler's 'Fonzie' (A.H. Fonzarelli) for classic 'cool'. The only real problem is getting to know what they are thinking. Commenting unnecessarily, and being reactionary is never 'cool'. Charisma, especially if enigmatic and mysterious will seem to conceal hidden depths. The façade rarely survives close examination.

Corporate Kids

These guys know how to survive and prosper in corporate jungles. They know the value of compliance and how to create the right impression in order to gain future security. If they keep their heads down, well below the parapet, they can avoid in-fighting and climb the corporate ladder unhindered. With shows of brilliance and putting the works of Nicoló Machiavelli into practice, they can attain a place on any board of directors.

Cranks?

Yes, it's true: some women want to eat their placenta after child-birth. Others quietly believe that aliens are already among us (how else could science have advanced so quickly in the last 120 years?). Others believe that shark fin extract and powdered rhino horn have medicinal value. Some believe that 'natural' is always better than 'synthetic' (they should try powering their car with 'natural', un-processed crude oil).

Some of those who express these ideas are psychotic; others are just ill-informed and would struggle to justi-fy their beliefs when cross-questioned about the science involved. Some are attention-seekers using controversy as their USB. Doctors will need to decide which type they are. Many are benign, so it might be best to respect their views and agree to differ. Politeness costs nothing, even though sometimes seen as a weakness.

Frustrated with 'standard' medical advice and a com-puter that always says 'NO', some will turn to faith healing and prayer. A significant number will benefit from the experience. I never expressed an objection to 'alternative' methods, especially if harmless and they brought comfort. Given that placebos help 20% of those who take them, the onus is firmly on the medical profession to achieve better results.

Some doctors see all alternate ideas as nonsense and will keep their engagement with the unscientific to a mini-mum. Any affront caused by their relaxation of scientif-ic rigour may need to be swallowed with a pinch of salt should a patient report a real improvement after using an alternative, unscientific method.

On occasions, I have been told by patients that I am not just a doctor, but 'a healer'. They are referring indirectly, of course, to my use of the art of medicine. I took this as a compliment. It is important to realise that there are many medically untrained people who, by their presence, improve how others feel. Some of their explanations about how they bring benefit can be mystical or pseudo-scientific, rather than scientific. Many doctors do not seen any of this as their brief. They have no wish to depart from scientific appraisal.

If introducing dogs onto hospital wards can benefit patients (animal-assisted therapy), what else might? If the idea helps, and there is no obvious harm to it, why object to interventions that will expand our scope of humanity? Doctors and nurses must always be prepared for the unexpected.

Practised well, the art of medicine requires one to know when to say something, when to say nothing, when to be accommodating, and when to be economical with the truth. Improving morale is not 'doing nothing'. Morale can affect morbidity and mortality, but questions of medical integrity can arise. In any personal clinical contest between maintaining professional integrity and improving patient morale, every doctor and nurse must take a position.

We should recognise that faith, even misplaced faith (in keeping with a growing anti-science movement), can act as a powerful adjunct to medical intervention. Because faith is a strongly held persuasion and offers a powerful influence, it would waste the time of doctors and nurses to try persuading some patients otherwise. Some patients will counter a scientific explanation by saying, 'you just don't understand spiritual matters'. Clearly, you may not have yet 'found the path', or 'seen the light'. Imagine the accolade that awaits any patient who can successfully persuade a doctor to follow their prescribed path to enlightenment.

In 1984, architect Carl Marsh came to consult me one evening. He was dressed for business in his three-piece suit. I asked why he had come, to be told, 'I've been sent'. 'Do you have heart disease?', I enquired. 'I do have an aortic valve problem, but that's not why I am here.', he replied. 'I have been sent to you to give you this book, but let me explain. I am an architect and a professional spiritual medium. I am a prison and have given a number of radio broadcasts on the subject. I knew you would not be ready to accept what I have to say so I brought you this book, written by a surgeon who discovered spirituality. It is called The Path of the Masters. Perhaps you will read it later in life.

Carl told me that he had had conversations with Moses, Jesus Christ and Mohammed, and had written a small book to help others understand the sprit world. He said that after dying with heart failure, who would no longer return to being human (implying that he would have attained a higher state of being).

When I examined him, a moderately severe aortic valve leakage was obvious. He needed further investigation, per-haps leading to valve replacement. He refused, saying, that prolonging his life was not what he wanted.

Carl was aware that he sounded delusional, and claimed not to be schizophrenic. Being highly plausible does not exclude it, though. I must leave my readers to come to their own conclusions.

Successful California surgeon, Dr. Julian P. Johnson, claimed to have 'been sent to India' to learn from gurus. He wrote, 'The Path of the Masters' (1939).

Criminals

Few patients will cause doctors and nurses to sense danger. The most troublesome are usually those who are economical with the truth; those who lie to get what they want, the devious and the downright criminal. These patients will test the resolve of doctors and nurses. They will bring any desire to help them into conflict with professional integrity.

I had a patient who lied about her role as a PA in a film production company. She feigned back pain and said that only tramadol helped her. I gave her a prescription for a small amount, but soon after, she returned and told me she had lost the prescription.

After that, several pharmacists reported dealing with falsified prescriptions. The most relevant descriptive word for her was 'plausible'. Like many practised criminals, they are composed, confident, and plausible; indistinguishable from most professionals, in fact. They are professional cheats, fraudsters, and liars.

I was alone one evening in my clinic when two men appeared, descending the stairs from the first floor (I learned later that they had stolen money from the dental suite). I remember how quietly confident and self-assured they were. 'We wanted to make a dental appointment', one claimed. 'At 8.30pm, long after office hours?' I asked. 'You never know your luck, do you?' one said nonchalantly as he walked out of the front door. The following morning, we discovered the extent of the burglary. In retrospect, I guess I was lucky not

*to have been threatened. I was alone, and could hardly
have defended myself against two strong young men.*

Those facing a Criminal Court appearance will sometimes say anything to get a doctor's support. They may
try to get a doctor to bear false witness. They need to
understand a doctor's role. In order to put them in the
picture, I said to one, 'I will help you as much as I
can, provide all the information I hold, but will never
lie on your behalf.' Rhetorically, I asked them: 'Why
would a doctor want to jeopardise his career by giving
a false statement?' I never met a criminal who didn't
immediately understand my position.

Some drug addicts and criminals will threaten doctors
if they do not satisfy their demands. These situations
are challenging. I was once told that I risked getting my
throat cut if I didn't help! Mostly, these are bullies; the
truly bad guys have no need to threaten or give warnings
of their action. *Courage mes braves!* Say 'NO' and mean
it. With luck, such patients will respect you. Involve
your colleagues; report them to the Police, and check
that your video surveillance cameras are working.

After being threatened, the police can be of less helpful than imagined. After all, no crime has been committed. To your dismay, they may imply that you should
return only after being assaulted; they will then have
an actual crime to deal with. Reporting a threat might
help if there is an outstanding arrest warrant against the
culprit.

*Criminals can be accused falsely if typecast. I remember one
such patient with an implanted defibrillator. Heart failure
(dilated cardiomyopathy) had caused him to have repeated*

episodes of ventricular tachycardia (VT). With left heart
failure, he was short of breath on minimal effort.

The prosecutor in court suggested that he had run 200 metres
holding a heavy iron bar intending to attack two athletic
young men. The allegation was that he had assaulted these
two young burglars after chasing them uphill.

When the judge asked me what I thought of the incident,
I suggested that such physical exertion would be beyond his
exercise ability. I went further and suggested that even ap-
pearing in court might prove a danger to him. Having had
several surprise defibrillator shocks, he was not keen to ex-
perience another. The prosecutor, whose desire it was to pro-
ceed with the case, suggested that we might, therefore, have
a resuscitation team standing by - just in case. The judge
looked me in the eye, and peering over his half-rim glasses,
said, 'Would you care to comment, Dr. Dighton?' I replied,
'I don't think I have heard a more inappropriate suggestion
made in court.' The judge agreed and dismissed the case.

Wheeler-dealers and criminals can offer financial re-
wards, or other inducements, if only a doctor will act to
help them avoid prosecution. Some convicted criminals are
among the most charming, intelligent, engaging and per-
suasive people one will meet. Not everyone will keep their
promises, but, paradoxically, most criminals will. Having
experienced the long arm of the law, criminals know better
than most, that good-will, loyalty, and keeping promises
are invaluable.

A young man once asked me if I could provide evidence
for what he claimed to be his pathological fear of needles.
After his arrest for drinking and driving, he had refused to
give a blood sample for an alcohol test (after a positive urine

alcohol test), at a police station. A neuroticism questionnaire (the MHQ, or Middlesex Hospital Questionnaire) suggested that he had high levels of anxiety. The result did not support any phobia, but it provided some evidence of his neurotic state. The court gave him the benefit of the doubt and discharged him. He later told me he had falsified the answers to my questionnaire. Surprise, surprise!

Dictator

This potentially dangerous sub-type of controller can be both arrogant and ignorant (see **ALBer**), they can seem disinterested in a doctor's opinion. They are demanding and purport to know best. They are only fleetingly in listening mode and may see it as a doctor's privilege to deal with them. The first problem is to find sense in their demands, and then to be as helpful as one can. If scolded, they will not usually return

Digital Beings

A product of the information age is 'the digital self'. Mobile phone apps can continuously record 'big data' – our respiratory rate, the number of steps taken, and our pulse rates. Collecting clinical data of doubtful clinical significance is one thing, accepting the growth of fashionable narcissism, is another. It is now fashionable to be narcissistic.

Doctors as Patients

Doctors are a special sub-group of patient, simply because they can decide what is wrong with them before asking for another opinion. A doctor consulting with another doctor must remain objective and independent, and take their patient's professional opinion seriously. Doctors as patients need to see that every clinical ritual is performed correctly, be it history taking or examination. Taking shortcuts and jumping to conclusions must be resisted. No doctor wants to be 'short-changed' clinically by another.

One must studiously await all the data before concluding one's thoughts. The confidence and trust of patients who are doctors will by earned more easily if the examining doctor behaves like their former lecturers and teachers – knowledgeable and respectful.

The diagnosis and management of other doctors must make complete clinical sense. Doctors, as patients, will have arguments that only special experience and specialised knowledge can counter. For a doctor to put their life in another doctor's hands, an adequate response must be given to their every challenge. One can only move forward with mutual agreement.

The patient may be a doctor, but they are also a patient, and need to be respected for both roles. Doctors will find it difficult to deal with doctors who are not comfortable with their role as patient. For one doctor to transfer clinical responsibility to another doctor is a big step.

When dealing with non-medical patients, many of us use infantile expressions like 'just pop on the couch', and 'can I feel your tummy?' Few would use such expressions when dealing with other doctors, so why use them at all?

Duper's Delight

Duping others may not be illegal, but is always fraudulent. This behaviour is common among drug addicts who will concoct any excuse to get the extra prescriptions they want. They will tell doctors they have lost their prescription, lost their pills, had them stolen, or eaten by their dog. Some will say that they feel more secure with lots of stock-piled drugs (for fear of running out); others will claim that they had to share them with a needy friend.

I must admit to being naïve: I mostly believed my patients (until proven otherwise). But then, if I had wanted to become a drug inspector, or work for the fraud squad, I would not have applied to medical school.

An ex-nurse and her husband both duped me. She was getting diazepam and zopiclone from both her GP and me, while swearing that I was the only one prescribing for her. I had warned her pharmacist and her GP of this possibility, seven years before, when I suspected she was double-dealing. I had her GP's agreement to be her sole prescriber. When her GP retired, whoever replaced him did not read my original letter detailing our agreement. I suspected as much when I inadvertently saw her coming out of her GP's surgery.

Later on, her GP records revealed she had been alternating between me and her new GP to get extra drugs. Without doubt, she had been duping me.

The case came before the MPTS (Medical Practitioner's Tribunal Service at the GMC). They held me accountable, not her NHS GP. They believed I had exposed her to risks beyond what her NHS GP, or an addiction specialist would have allowed. The patient never came to any harm in my hands, with twice weekly visits over a seven-year period and drug doses that never escalated. At no time did she make an allegation against me; the complaint came from a pharmacist. The boring but important details are in my book, 'The NHS. Our Sick Sacred Cow'.

WARNING. Being deceived by a patient can lead doctors and nurses to be classed as unfit to practice. It has not helped the doctor-patient relationship for doctors and nurses to have become suspicious of every patient.

The Fearful

Many patients feel anxious while consulting doctors. They may be shy, or have a genuine fear about what may transpire during the consultation. Putting patients at ease is a valuable interpersonal skill and a clinical art. Patients will remain buttoned up and communicate poorly if their fear and anxiety is not eased.

Interesting People

Many of my patients were interesting people. Like many other doctors, I had side-interests: research, writing, travel, finance, art, music, etc. Many of my patients knew much more about these subjects than I did, so I found it interesting and informative to talk to them.

As experienced travellers, some of my patients could provide me with excellent travel advice.

My daughter Anna once travelled to Venice on a school trip. One of my patients (Franco Dorili) knew the restaurant director at the Cipriani Hotel on Giudecca Island. 'I will

*telephone him for you, and book a table for her', he said. 'I
will ask him to take special care of her.' And so he did.*

*I asked my patient Colin Fitch where I should eat in New
York. He booked me a table at the River Café, just below
Brooklyn Bridge overlooking Manhattan – just to make
sure I had a waterside table.*

*When I asked Alan Reed where to stay in San Francisco, he
arranged the Fairmont Hotel for me, on a floor high enough
to see the bay and Alcatraz.*

Many patients 'in the know' were generous to me with
their time and knowledge. Many took pleasure in advising
me. The mutual sharing of beneficial knowledge is an act
of friendship. This is one pleasure to be found while practising traditional pastoral medicine. It contrasts with the
rigid and formal style of practices focused on nothing but
disease (albeit the most important of issues).

If medical school selection committees continue to seek
only high grade, detached scientists as applicants, the traditional pastoral role of doctors will diminish. A broader
based education and extensive life experiences, were once
prerequisites for all would-be doctors, especially if their
ambition was to provide pastoral care. Selection committees may not be sympathetic to 60-year-old ideas. It would
never do for them to be classed as 'old fashioned', or to
admit that 'once upon a time' our predecessors were just as
wise as we, and knew more about how to practise than we
do now. The way doctors deal with patients has changed
little, but the politics has never stood still.

There is another way to make pastoral care acceptable.
Re-brand it, and call it 'social prescribing'.

Gamers

In his book, '*The Games People Play*', (1964), Eric Berne describes the gaming aspects of human relationships. Patients playing interpersonal games want to win by scoring points of advantage. The scoring of points allows the declaration of winners and losers. Some patients try to involve medical professionals in their games.

Many have attempted to draw me into their attention-seeking games with partners. Someone who might wish to test their partner's interest, respect or love, might try to test them by creating medical concern. They might choose to present with symptoms calculated to draw attention to their health, and the more puzzling the better. The patient's partner, or ex-partner, might then take the bait and show concern. Their concern might lead to demanding second and third opinions, or suggesting further tests to confirm the diagnosis. They might suggest a change of doctor if not enough interest is shown, or if the diagnosis seems ill-considered, or too benign. There is a hidden point to the process. The payoff for the patient is to get to know just how much their partner really cares for them.

Berne had a lot to say about alcoholism; he regarded it as a potentially lethal, three-handed 'game'. The players in the game are the alcoholic, the uncompromising one who is unsympathetic, and the 'patsy' – the helpful one. All three must interrelate for alcoholism to continue. Some alcoholics can feel so dejected they might commit suicide. After dying, surely that will make the uncompromising ones, feel guilty. The intended message was: 'That will teach you. You should have taken me seriously.' To help understand their role in the 'game' of alcoholism, psychotherapy can provide insights for each player. The question then is, will such insight help to bring about any beneficial change?

If doctors are lucky enough to practise medicine with extensive personal knowledge of their patients, their family and work colleagues, getting drawn into inter-personal games becomes either less likely or easily possible. By recognising the dynamics, one can either play along (if it will benefit your patient), or take no part. Doctors must recognise as soon as possible, every attempt made to involve them in attention-seeking, and other manipulative games patients want to play.

GG: Good Guys

Most patients are pleasant, fair, respectful, diplomatic and reasonable. Grace and charm are rarer virtues. They mostly display 'good behaviour', not easily corrupted by NBW's (nasty bits of work). It is easy to define good behaviour. It is that which leaves everyone in their midst feeling comfortable. Good guys are usually obvious from the very first meeting.

Matthew C was a happy 5-year-old in 2016. We instantly got on. His mother told me that whenever they passed my clinic, Mat would want to call in and say 'Hello'. The last time he called in, he gave me a hug and a kiss on the cheek. He may have only been five years old, but he was already a GG.

Grammar School, Comprehensive, or Public School?

A patient's level and type of education can influence their medical management. Peer group influences, attitudes, and general behaviour patterns of patients can undoubtedly influence the doctor-patient relationship. (see more comment under 'Doctors and Nurses as Characters').

Hopeful Patients

Patients have many and various attitudes towards disease: 'It's not fair.'; 'I can beat this.'; 'Why me?'; 'I don't do illness.' Others are fatalistic and will take whatever comes.

Even when doing the job well, doctors and nurses will always find a limit to what each patient will allow them to do. It can depend on how well we inform them, and how much we involve them in the decision-making process. The art of medicine requires that we know our patient well enough to gauge the amount of information they can handle. Patients are right to use their experience of their previous consultations, appraisals and judgements to assess the value of a doctor or nurse. An accolade I once received from a patient was: 'I will never act on any medical advice until I get your advice.' This resulted from him comparing my opinions to those he received from other doctors. For high levels of trust like this to be built with patients, a few lengthy, tried and tested, clinical interventions must have taken place.

The need for hope is universal, but varies a lot between patients. Prayer and hope can both influence prognosis. For some doctors, this subject lies over the hills, and far, far away from their focus; often too far over the event horizon for a blinkered scientific mind to handle. The scientific method, as the Holy Grail of science, attracts the same passion among some doctors as any religion, so they should respect the vital nature of belief and faith to some patients.

Zeus's vengeance package contained many evils, including death. They all escaped into the world after Pandora opened her jar (not a box). After closing it, only 'Elpis' (hope or expectation) remained. For some patients, this will be all they have left. There are reasons some hopes need to be dashed, and others left in place. Knowing patients well will usually guide doctors to the best course of action. With so many immeasurable inter-personal considerations, there can be no legitimate place for fixed rules or algorithmic thinking. There should always be a place for hope, compassion, empathy, dedication, goodwill, and some respect for faith and belief.

My uncle Charlie came to see me with a DVT and painful thrombophlebitis. He had been a smoker, and a chest x-ray had revealed a hilar mass (lung cancer). 'Whatever I have wrong with me,' he said, 'I want you to deal with it. You don't need to share the details with me. If you want me to have a test, or a treatment, I will do whatever you think best. I want to delegate my management to you.'

In the early 1970s, the average prognosis of squamous cell carcinoma of the lung, after lobectomy and radiotherapy, was 6 months and one day. Without treatment, it was six months. I told his son, who agreed with me, that giving him a cancer diagnosis would adversely affect him psychologically. I elected not to tell him his diagnosis, and not to get

*him treated. I wanted to preserve his lifestyle without the
burden of fear and anxiety. News of a poor prognosis would
have devastated him, so we kept it to ourselves. His only
treatment was anticoagulation. Despite the poor prognosis,
he lived asymptomatically for three years before he died.*

Knowledge alone is not enough. Clinical experience
must distil what knowledge we have into wisdom. Wise
clinical judgement is universally available, but is useful
only when applied appropriately to an individual patient.
The ability to make such judgements and to know their
proper application, defines a competent physician. The
ability to comply with every fixed rule, and guideline, regardless of clinical appropriateness, may define a compliant knowledgeable doctor, but not always one who is fully
competent. The ability to comply with every regulation is
not a qualification for clinical perspicacity.

*In the 17ᵗʰ century, Nicholas Culpepper, the apothecary, said
that patients attended his practice in Spitalfields (London)
to get an injection of hope.*

Hope is good, but reconnaissance, planning, and vali-
dation will often prove more successful.

The Incapable

If a patient lacks the mental capacity to remember facts,
or to process information, he might be unable to engage
in medical decision-making processes. The list of causes is long, but includes intoxication, delirium (related to
physical illness), dementia, cerebral underdevelopment or
damage, together with psychoses (being out of touch with
reality). It can also apply to those suffering extreme stress;
it is difficult to cope with problems when pre-occupied.

All need safeguarding and support. Most will need someone they would trust to decide on their behalf, acting in their best interests. This subject requires its own treatise.

Influencers

They do not exist on TikTok and Instagram alone. Family, friends, the internet, floor-cleaners and fellow patients, sometimes influence hospital patients more than doctors and nurses.

When patients shared Nightingale wards, I once overheard a post-op patient speaking to a pre-op patient about their surgeon they shared: 'I wish you luck with the operation, mate. His patients rarely do well.'

Interrogators

There are those who enjoy interrogating others, even when the matters concerned are trivial. They have an obsessional need to delve into the detail. A summary response will not satisfy them. Getting all the facts is essential to their enquiries, even with inconsequential, everyday matters. Dealing with them requires patience and tolerance. Doctors and nurses will need tact to bring their interrogation to an end.

IS: Internet Savvy

Incorrect information can be worse than no information, so doctors and nurses should encourage patients to corroborate what they have learned. The savvy patient may think he knows it all, especially after consulting 'Dr. Google'. With an unbalanced opinion, based on cherry-picked information, he may well have decided what he needs from a doctor. He is unlikely to have a considered picture of his problem. Only a few will have enough experience, knowledge, or judgement to assess the validity and relevance of the medical 'facts' they gleaned from the internet. Regardless of this, some patients will reach correct conclusions. Given that most people will refer to the internet after being given a diagnosis, it might be best to provide them with the best search terms.

Steve came to see me with his wife. His extensive research led him to believe that she had Lyme disease. In the end, the diagnosis proved correct. Well done, Steve. All patients deserve to be listened to, and given the benefit of the doubt.

Patient demands arise from many situations, the most valid of which is ill-health and personal suffering. There are other sources of demand, like media outlets promoting a sensational new medical advance. For doctors, the many unproven 'advances', 'cures', and 'tests', described by the media, can find doctors having to explain the need for double-blind controlled experiments. Few patients are trained to distinguish between codswallop and well-conducted research.

When doctors dismiss new ideas, patients may take it as unsympathetic, overbearing, and unhelpful. A patient's insistence that, 'there must be something to it. Why else would anyone publish it?' can seem churlish to deny. Even with verified facts, they may remain unconvinced, and simply go elsewhere. Only after they deteriorate will some patients question the wisdom of following a strategy suggested by the media. Freedom of choice has consequences.

When researching the side-effects of drugs, or the work of a doctor, patients can get distorted ideas. After all, who can claim to be exact in assessing probability and risk, when choosing anything? In order to inspire confidence, I sometimes used simple examples from my experience. I might say: 'In thirty years of using this drug, I never saw this, or that side-effect.' Alternatively, I might say: 'In my experience, half of those taking these drugs experience muscle discomfort. Even with personal recommendations, patient bias can be difficult to overcome.

Kidnappers and Hijackers

I met with a patient of mine, Mr. P, while in Istanbul. He invited me to his flat the next day for afternoon tea. Mr. P and his wife greeted me, together with eight of their relatives they had assembled to get my advice. The further west and north a doctor goes in Europe, the less this is likely to happen.

Some hijackers are polite: *'I know you're on holiday, doctor, but I wonder if I could trouble you for a moment?'*

If a doctor is someone who flies a lot, or takes cruises or holidays on small islands, he will be at risk of getting medically hijacked. Someone sitting by the pool, at a bar, or at the same table during meals, may not resist seeking a medical opinion. In a diminishing number of cultures, doctors are still demigods. And, how often does one meet a demigod? Meeting one is an opportunity too good to be true, and not to be missed.

Most people expect doctors and nurses to be kind and helpful. Desist! These anonymous 'patients' will rarely appreciate the difficulty you will have basing an opinion on their history alone. Be prepared for scorn if you don't comply with their request, and expect anger when they feel rejected.

Some will try repeatedly to interest you in their *'once upon a time'* medical misadventure; they will even draw their friends and partners into the discussion, just to provide corroboration. For the sake of a little added drama, their evidence will often include details of just how close they came to death. Some will contend that no doctor before has ever really listened to them; not like you. How lucky they were to survive, and how lucky to have met you.

There is no easy or courteous way to fend them off, unless you follow the example of one well-known celebrity. When asked by a fellow traveller if he was Joe Bloggs, he replied, 'Not to-day, I'm not!' This will only shake off the least determined; a less considerate, insensitive or stronger form of rebuke will be required for the more ardent.

None of this applies to me. I have always been far too soft to deny any medical hijacker. Rebuking others in need is a cultural issue for me. My parents raised me to be respectful. I also believe that having medical knowledge and the talent to use it, comes with a sovereign duty: to help others medically, whenever one can. If as a doctor or nurse, altruism is not your thing, travel completely *in cognito*. Tell nobody what it is you do, or suffer consequences that may not be to your liking. Personally, I have never found it a problem.

Although rare in the UK, there are countries where it is usual to be invited to join a club, team, or firm as a recognised clique member. Within the clique, there might be a free exchange of information, goodwill, goods, meals, hotel stays, and other services. I am a member of one such Cypriot clique (of very close friends and associates). My role within the group is medical adviser; not because I want to exchange my advice for good will, meals or hotel stays, but because my friends need my support and guidance when they deal with their doctors. I get the benefit of their support in all worldly matters.

Kind and Genteel

These patients can make a doctor feel that their work is worthwhile. See also: OK, and GG.

Lazy Buggers

I have always been too polite to say it, but would like to have asked the occasional colleague or patient, 'When did your last servant die?' Some people have been so spoilt, having always had their every wish granted, they expect everyone to serve them. Some were born idle, and some have had idleness thrust upon them; others developed their lazy ways after learning just how easy it is to get 'friends' to step in and help.

Feigning illness and false incapacity are both ploys some will use to attract sympathetic helpers. Watch out for false gratitude and fluttering eyelashes. One can easily get hooked by the idle and the undeserving. Curb their demands at the earliest stage.

Liars

One third of us lie every day.
Richard Wiseman. Psychologist.

I always had a major weakness with my outlook to patients: I believed most of what they told me. I never found it too much of a problem, except for being duped three times in fifty-three years. The last incident led to my suspension (by the Medical Practitioners Tribunal Service, October 2019). It did not shake my trust in patients, only my trust in regulators. (Read about it in my book, '*The NHS. Our Sick Sacred Cow*').

Unlike Pinocchio, human noses don't grow as lies are told. Doctors and nurses must understand the reasons for patients lying. One is to avoid any corruption of their self-image ('nothing wrong with me doc.'), another is to avoid unpleasant consequences ('if I tell the truth, doctors might do some nasty tests'). With drug addicts, lying about having lost their prescription is a common ploy used to get extra drugs. The consequences of lying can, of course, be tragic. Some patients fear illness and suffering so much, they would sooner lie and be dead than suffer. They need counselling.

There is a growing linguistic science being used to detect lies. Analysis of recorded interviews given before criminal trials by those eventually convicted, has led to the identification of many reliable verbal indicators of lying.

MAE: Mental Age of Eight

When asked, a medical colleague of mine agreed to write memos for insurance company employees. After this experience, his advice to me was simple: when writing to instruct corporate staff, assume they all have a mental age of eight years; the majority will then understand your memos. He had no intention to insult any eight-year-old child.

'Against ignorance, the Gods strive in vain.'
Friedrich Schiller (1801)

Manipulators

There are those whose *modus operandi* is to barter and
make deals. If they present as patients, their priority may
not be medical at all, it may be to make a proposal or to
certificate their 'good standing'. Their quest is to profit
somehow, like getting you or your staff to make all their
appointments for them. If you make an appointment for
them (after many telephone calls going backwards and
forwards), they might try something extra. They might ask
you to confirm that they will not have to wait too long.
This all sounds bizarre, but it happens. Such patients want
unpaid servants. Business gurus regard them as effective
delegators; I regard them as users.

A manipulator will first try to get a doctor on his side.
'We've been friends for so long, haven't we?' is their common opening gambit. Translated into motivational terms,
there is a tacit threat here: 'surely, you wouldn't want to
risk losing me as a friend?' He wins if you give him the
recognition he seeks, or if (in private practice) you waive
your fees (friends don't charge friends, do they?). In the
NHS, where direct payment is not required (except for
signing passports / certificates, etc.), some patients will try
to obligate their doctor. If you become obligated, they
will try to use you, and your time, whenever they want.
They will want favours, with no thought of reciprocation,
whether it be for goodwill or an agreement to follow your
advice. Right from the start, their behaviour should signal
caution.

If they don't get what they want, they can turn nasty and be disapproving. That is why some doctors need to 'man-up' and refuse to bend to their will, right from the start. They will get upset once they realise we are not all pushovers. Beware, though, manipulators are nimble; they will deftly change their tactics and demands. They will quickly try alternative approaches: a new deal or a new understanding between friends.

'No' is a word unacceptable to manipulators. The word 'No' has a cultural perspective. In Russian culture, it means 'not negotiable': 'Nyet' means 'No', not 'perhaps', or I'll think about it. In British, Greek and some eastern cultures, 'No' is often just an early step in the process of negotiation.

If you prove useful, a manipulator will tell all his associates how soft and amenable you are as a doctor. You could become the 'go to' person. Manipulators will not support you in a crisis, and will be the first to blame you when things go wrong. Beware of manipulators, unless you are shrewder than them and can spot one from afar. Unfortunately, most manipulators are street-wise, and that usually means they are streets ahead of most doctors and nurses.

Martyrs

These are easy to spot. Their behaviour means: *'I am suffering, and nobody can help me now. It's my destiny to suffer.'*

In the film *'The Life of Brian'* (1979), a Roman prisoner (played by Michael Palin) had been hanging upside-down in his cell for years. For the sake of satire, he says that the Romans who put him there were actually quite reasonable. In fact, he felt obliged to them for being so 'fair' and understanding. A happy martyr indeed.

MASH: Mad **AS** a **H**atter

These patients have ideas that will not only cause doctors to raise an eyebrow, but will cause some to be aghast with incredulity. Among them are attention seekers and conspiracy theorists. Some are delusional, others are misguided with opinions developed mostly from information, cherry picked to suit their purpose.

MASHs are not alone in their cherry-picking ability. Those who employ meta-analyses to analyse multiple drug trials, need to be adept cherry-pickers (a common source of error in 'evidence-based medicine'). The selection criteria applied to any study group, will limit the clinical relevance of the research (cherry-picked) to that group alone. Doctors must always scrutinise research selection criteria for any match to their patients. This subject is essential for every doctor who wants to put research results into practice.

MOMA and POPA

Mater **O**h **MA**ter (Matriach), or **P**ater **O**h **PA**ter (Patriarch). These patients have taken their entire family (support group, or work group) under their wing, and under their control. It is essential to know whether they are acting in a beneficial or a malign way. Once there is proof of a doctor's worth, it is they who will direct their family members to them for advice. They are few in number, but are all well worth identifying. It is always useful to identify the Top Guy, or Head Honcho (*Ganze Macher*).

Neanderthal (*Homo neanderthalensis*)

Although thought extinct, some of their characteristics survive. Homo sapiens will have bred with them, guaranteeing the survival of some of their supposed characteristics: physical strength, resistance to cold, physical endurance, and perhaps lower intelligence (relative to Homo sapiens – the wise man – that is).

Neurotic and TFBF – Too Fussy by Far

Many patients make clinically insignificant observations (in a doctor's opinion), that will nevertheless concern them. They might think that every naevus is a melanoma, or every headache the first sign of a brain tumour. If they are obsessional, they will test everybody's patience. The fear, anxiety, hysteria, and hypochondriasis experienced by any TFBF patient needs sympathetic handling. They can learn the real clinical significance of their concerns through education, and with cognitive therapy they can learn to face their worst fears. These patients can consume a lot of consultation time. If doctors don't have enough of it, they must refer them.

A surrogate TFBF situation exists. Here, a third party does the fussing, often to the embarrassment of the patient. Minders will bring patients to you, like dogs on a lead. The minder (mother, father, friend) will tell you the story, while the patient remains silent. While this is a common situation when dealing with children, it also occurs with adults. It is quite easy to deal with, as long as the discussion includes the patient from the start. Some minders are devious manipulators, and should be side-lined; others deserve honour for their genuine concern and involvement.

If there are any psychiatrists or psychologists reading what follows, I must apologise for the simplification. My aim is to provide a simple guide to neurotic traits.

The Crisp-Crown Index grades each of six psychoneurotic traits as average, less than average or greater than average (*Middlesex Hospital Questionnaire* (MHQ), B.J.Psychiatry (1966); 112: 917-23). The six traits are *anxiety, depression, obsession, hysteria, phobia and hypochondriasis*. They will all be obvious clinically to physicians when they are well developed.

In the minimally expressed, stoic state, they can be difficult to detect. A stoic non-neurotic state is typical of pilots, astronauts, and Victoria Cross holders; they have a matter-of-fact attitude to life, not an emotional one. Clinically, this makes them easier to deal with.

Those with a well-developed obsessional trait (nit-pickers with attention to detail) do well in jobs that require meticulousness. The same trait can prove exhausting to the doctors and nurses who have to deal with them. Their obsessional trait can be of psychiatric significance. I once met a patient who insisted on sweeping the autumn leaves from her front path, in a strong wind at 2am in the morning.

Brian Bridgman was a chief helicopter pilot instructor, with 4000 hours of flying experience. He managed every detail of his life precisely. He was always in control. Consultations with him were always succinct and to the point. 'I have three problems to-day', he would say. We discussed them briefly, and he would then summarise his understanding of our conversation. He then detailed how he would implement the actions we agreed.

Brian died in January (2016) flying his helicopter from Scotland to Kent, after it developed a fatal turbine bearing failure. His life ended because of a mechanical failure that was entirely beyond his control.

I used the MHQ for many decades, and computerised it (a DOS based, Dbase2 database program). I ran tests on over 1000 patients. After a while, feedback from the test allowed me to diagnose the six neurotic traits more easily. I found the questionnaire most useful for confirming depression and sub-clinical depression. The questionnaire was also useful for semi-quantifying anxiety (slight – average – severe). The information helped me appreciate the psychological state of patients, and its likely contribution to their clinical state. This was often of relevance to planning their future medical management.

I had an occasion to speak with both Crisp and Crown. They were both rather surprised that anyone was still using their 1960s questionnaire, so long after they published it. Useful techniques do not degrade with age and may not need to be superseded. Fashion and technical advances alone will dictate when this happens.

Here is an example of an unexpected response from a patient with both high anxiety and hypochondriasis (somatic anxiety) scores.

Mary was 68-years-old. She had been complaining about feeling unwell for years. She was also complaining that her husband took no interest in her condition. All her symptoms were nonspecific, and several general examinations had revealed nothing of diagnostic value.

Then I tested her urine and found blood (microscopic haematuria). I told her I had found something, but probably nothing of significance. I asked her for an early morning specimen. That showed the same trace of blood. To this news she said: 'Thank God you've found something wrong, doctor. Everyone thinks I am an incurable hypochondriac.' An IVP (we used intravenous pyelograms at the time to opacify the urinary tract with an iodine-based contrast dye), showed a non-functioning left kidney. Cancer, was my first thought. An operation revealed something else - a left renal (kidney) abscess. The infection had destroyed her kidney completely. It had become a bag of pus, which must have affected her health for many years. This explained why she had felt so unwell for so long.

There is a moral to the tale. Doctors should always take extra care with patients labelled 'hypochondriac'. The simple fact is that no hypochondriac is exempt from physical disease.

No Entiendo?

Doctors will sometimes see a patient's facial expression change to one of incomprehension, while they try to explain technical details. Some will signal with a glazed look, meaning 'I have zoned-out'; 'you've lost me'. Perhaps they have they not understood what was said? Is nothing sinking in? Might they be pre-occupied? Perhaps they have already decided what they want and anything you say will be irrelevant.

If your message is important enough, ask them to repeat it back to you, and get them to recall the instructions you gave them. Be prepared to conclude that you have wasted your breath.

In a high-profile case (Chester v Afshar, 14.10. 2004), neurosurgeon Mr. Fary Afshar, a medical school contemporary of mine, said he had warned his patient about the complications of laminectomy (inter-vertebral disc removal; she had several prolapsed discs). The patient later sustained neurological damage and claimed that he had not warned her fully of the possible complications.

The House of Lords decided that a doctor's failure to inform a patient fully of every surgical risk vitiates the need to show that harm would follow from failing to inform.

If litigation against doctors gathers any further momentum, we will need to video every consultation.

OK Patients

These sensible patients are both compliant and understanding. They listen, understand, and ask pertinent questions. They learn easily and can decide what to do in their best interest.

Objective

These patients are usually reliable historians. History taking is easy with patients who are intelligent, objective, succinct, and have an excellent memory. One can handle them efficiently if their narrative composition is concise (rather than lengthy, and 'once upon a time'). Often, though, there will be a need to clarify what a patient says, and what it is they mean to say.

Obligators

See 'manipulators'. If doctors or nurses ever accept a favour from a patient, they will be at risk of becoming obligated, although in my experience very few patients who give favours intend any obligation.

PITA: Pain In The Arse.

These patients are usually obsessional and must get what they want before they can move on. Those with some insight into being 'a pain in the arse', are no better, so strong is their obsessional trait. If a patient lacks insight into their annoying trait, doctors must make accurate notes of their demands, taking care that their words and punctuation are correct. PITA patients can waste a lot of a doctor's time, and put a strain on their affability, reasonableness, and sanity. There is another side to this coin. Their attention to detail can save their life, especially when they remind doctors of what they have overlooked.

Range Riders

Many patients become concerned when told that some of their laboratory results are not 'within normal limits' or are outside the normal range. In my practice, most of my patients wanted to be involved in their diagnosis and management so this is something which will take time to explain.

To explain what 'normal range' means, and the relevance of laboratory error, can be challenging. There is a difference between a variant of normal and a pathological result. Repeat testing for verification may be needed. Many will be happy only when their results are 'within normal limits'.

Patients self-recording their blood pressure has significantly contributed to the control of hypertension, even if taking it frightens some enough to cause high readings. Just as often it consoles them once they understand just how variable blood pressure can be. Quantitative measures of exercise undertaken, cigarettes smoked, pizzas eaten, and alcohol consumed, can all help clinical risk assessment (although patients often underestimate the quantities they consume). The errors involved in such data collection and their interpretation will concern only a few patients.

Recalcitrant Recidivists

'Can an Ethiopian change his skin or the leopard his spots?'
Jeremiah 13:23

Consider this contention: *there are many who repeatedly have strokes, heart attacks, and asthma attacks, because they continually (choose to) put up with unacceptable circumstances brought about by limited resources, an inappropriate sense of responsibility, and inappropriate loyalty or duty to others.*

The question is why would someone want to put their hand in a fire repeatedly, knowing that it will burn them each time? Some blame necessity; others will do it because they are brave, selfless, and able to take what comes whenever helping others. Despite the potential damage, the reasons for such sacrifice can be noble and intelligent. Others will repeatedly self-harm because they have yet to receive enough attention. Some have no wish to learn, and others cannot learn.

Some who know themselves to be allergic to nuts, will decide to eat one, just to see if they can get away with it. Others will buy feather pillows (they are softer), knowing that they are allergic to feathers. When agreeing to relate to someone as a partner, some will choose the same type of person each time, even though that led to previous relationship failures. Criminals carry on shop-lifting, and patients carry on drinking, taking drugs, and stressing themselves, hoping to get away with it. Some continue with the same behaviour despite their experiences of the likely consequences. Psychopaths (personality disorder), are an exception: they rarely care about consequences.

Over many decades, I told many patients to reduce their excessive alcohol intake, just to prove any adverse connection between their drinking and their hypertension. What did most do? You guessed it: they carried on drinking. Criminals are not the only ones who exhibit recidivist behaviour; the stupid, the driven, the obligated, and the addicted do it as well. This behaviour is so common one must regard it as 'usual' if not normal. Sometimes it is attention seeking, and part of an interpersonal game.

In order to change recidivist behaviour, many will need to gain some insight into reality, and be able to accept advice from one who has experienced the consequences. Group therapy will help some. This makes biological sense, since survival always depends on seeing things the way they really are; relying on fantasy is unreliable and too dangerous.

My guess is that we inherit the value we each place on insight. There those who can learn from their mistakes and those who cannot. From both evolutionary and clinical points of view, this feature is significant. A patient's insight into their medical condition, and the appropriateness and necessity of some clinical interventions, can influence their prognosis.

The Resentful

Resentment is one of the most powerful causes of steady personal decline, causing emotional instability, depression and aggression. Many who hold it will voice statements like, *'if it wasn't for you (him, them, it), I would be XYZ by now'.* Sometimes it is completely justified.

Some falsely blame others for not achieving their goals, whether it be fame, fortune or happiness. They will blame their parents, friends, business associates, spouses, and partners for their failure, and only rarely blame themselves. Resentment consumes energy through rumination and can adversely affect medical conditions as diverse as sleep disorder, immunity, migraine, IBS, psoriasis and angina.

Resentment is stressful because it consumes an excess of cerebral and physical energy (catecholamine, or adrenaline-like production). Many psychotherapists earn a good living, trying to help patients overcome their resentment. As an important medical issue, it can affect the natural history of many medical conditions.

Rich, Famous and Conceited

Being star-struck is for patients, not for doctors and nurses. Obsequiousness is out of place, whoever the patient. There is no need to comment further, except to issue a warning: watch out for patients who consider themselves too precious to commune with ordinary mortals. Their demands may prove unacceptable.

Mr. C. owned a nationwide chain of shops. One day he arrived at my clinic with an entourage that included three minders. At the time he arrived, my waiting room was unusually full (a rare occurrence). I could not drop everything and see Mr. C. immediately, so he left in a huff never to return.

His business office was enormous and had an over-sized desk placed on a dais. He had two minders always in attendance, standing on either side. From this elevated position, he could peer down onto his business associates sitting some distance away on an uncomfortable chair. In this way, he subordinated them before any word was spoken.

Self-Promotional Protagonist: SPP

If you want to sell lots of merchandise, hire a crowd to stand outside your shop. The crowd will attract inquisitive shoppers. If you want your restaurant to get busy, pay people to queue outside; it will soon be 'THE place' to be (as long as the price, and quality of food is acceptable).

There are patients and doctors who have sufficient charisma and ability to maximise their image (now referred to as their brand). They draw the attention of others and easily attract interest in their business practices or research. Unfortunately, disease has no respect for charisma. After achieving fame, dying young may be the only career move that might guarantee posthumous fame.

Making a noticeable fuss will help a patient grab the attention of medical staff, whether or not it is justified clinically. For those who need attention, and who are not demonstrative enough, dire consequences can follow.

I had several talkative patients who, when sitting in my reception area, could not resist telling others how wonderful a doctor I was. Another patient, himself a self-promoter, accused me of hiring people to sit in my waiting room for promotional purposes.

Selfish and Greedy

There are those with little regard for others who insist on being dealt with first, regardless of any medical priority. Unfortunately, it is selfish, dominant behaviour that succeeds most in drawing the attention of others.

Relatives and friends can display selfish, dominant behaviour on a patient's behalf. I have known this save a patient's life when they were being ignored.

I once visited a pregnant patient in labour. Although the chart showed the foetal heart rate dropping, nobody seemed too bothered. I suggested that a nurse should make an urgent call to whoever was on duty; a caesarean section needed to be considered. The SpR who arrived, agreed with me, and told me that nobody had informed him of the situation.

The brother of a female Nigerian patient brought his sister to see me. He told me this was a last ditch manoeuvre for her, and said, 'If you cannot cure her (of schizophrenia), we will take her into the jungle and leave her there!' As a Nigerian Chief, and head of the family, he could make that decision. He had brought her to the UK as a last resort, all local interventions having failed. I referred her to a psychiatrist, but never learned what happened to her.

SELPO: SELf-POssessed.

To know them is to understand conceit, vanity and narcissism.

JB (who had played the lead role in a successful film) said he couldn't sleep. He awoke each night, thinking that he was just imagining his role in the film. 'I Google myself to see if I am real - then I can relax', he said when interviewed.

Googling oneself is now a form of narcissism. It is certainly easier than finding a shady grove where lies 'a pool of silver-bright water' in which to see one's reflection (Metamorphoses; Ovid: Bk III:402-436).

SHUBE: Sentient HUman BEing.

These patients are a constant pleasure to help, and to be with.

Simple Folk

To survive modern life we all need to be street-wise to some extent. Being learned is unnecessary. In fact, being learned can unnecessarily complicate life. Simple, less educated folk, have no need for a complicated view of life; they will usually have less muddled thought, and will easily see the wood for the trees. Like Mr. Wilkins Micawber, in Dicken's *David Copperfield*, they will have learned one arithmetic lesson well: how to subtract one number from another. They are thus able to subtract their income from their expenditure. The result according to Mr. Wilkins Micawber will be happiness or misery. Meanwhile, the educated can pass their time performing statistical and Fourier analyses, and writing books.

Slobs

Unkempt, smelly, unwashed people all have a story to tell. In the bygone days of doctor's house visits, the decrepit state of some homes amazed me. Not all those living in squalor were poor. An unkempt state can indicate an eccentric personality, but it can also result from dejection, rejection, demoralisation or a psychiatric disorder.

Harry Enfield, in his comic TV portrayal of 'The Slobs' (BBC 2, 1990), showed that even winning the Lottery may not change their personal standards. Slobs may swap their plastic toilet seats for gold-plated ones, but their personal hygiene standards can remain unchanged.

One old, much debated social chestnut remains in dispute. The question is, do slobs make slums, or do slums make slobs? Both of my grandmothers lived in Victorian terraced houses in the East-End of London. Both had an answer to this anthropological question, although neither would have considered it a question worthy of consideration. One of them once said, 'everyone can afford soap'. Both scrubbed their front steps and pavement down to the curb. Their action went beyond personal pride; they showed civic pride.

The primary role of healthcare workers is not to judge people but to help them, especially those who cannot help themselves. Although it can suggest a psychiatric disorder, mental incapacity, or physical disability, incapacity can just as commonly relate to laziness or to drug and alcohol use. Coping with stress can cause the disintegration of self-care. Many of those who suffer the effects of stress will not function normally; some need urgent help. Others are happy and content to remain dishevelled, and see no reason to change.

When a methylated spirit (methyl alcohol) drinking vagrant died on the street, outside the London Hospital, in East London, the pathologists working there would correctly guess their former drinking status. At post-mortem, 'meth's drinkers' had liver damage, but arteries that were completely free of atherosclerosis ('furring'); just like the arteries of a baby. Despite this, I have never recommended methyl alcohol as a substitute for 'statin' drugs!

Smiling Depressives

Some people are humorous by nature and will laugh and joke even while depressed. They can smile when scared to death or troubled by bad news.

Spies and Intruders

Just occasionally, inquisitive or jealous doctors, will get their friends and relatives to spy on any competition.

It can happen if they are jealous of another doctor's success. Doctors and nurses can expect telephone calls and visits from potential patients searching for information. If anyone, including a doctor is successful, others might want to steal their intellectual property.

It used to happen to me occasionally, so I trained my staff to recognise spies. Medical spies give themselves away by using medical jargon; by being too knowledgeable, and by probing too deep. They will always avoid giving their name and contact details, since they will not want to be checked on. To confirm their suspicions while dealing with a telephone enquiry, my staff would ask them a direct question: 'For whom are you spying?' The question often brought about a little spluttering, and an abrupt end to the telephone call.

Our regulators sanction spying on doctors. In 2019, I pressed a senior, legally qualified CQC inspector, to confirm that they had sanctioned spying on me. She sheepishly admitted that they employed 'agencies' to collect information.

These 'agencies' made many telephone calls to check whether I was continuing to see non-cardiac patients after I had stopped providing a private general medical service (December 2018). A CQC GP Inspector, who had not long before visited my practice, made a follow-up telephone call posing as a cardiac patient. He said he had chest pain and asked my cardiac technician for advice. The CQC obviously questioned our ability to provide sound cardiac advice for symptomatic patients. Although tiresome, she played along. What these callers did not know was that we always recorded their telephone numbers. We would then return their calls. Their squirming denials of spying were always amusing.

It might stagger some patients to know that there are many medical bureaucrats who have little respect the doctors entrusted with the lives of patients. Their bureaucratic position entitles them to disbelieve doctors and nurses, and to consider them incompetent until proven otherwise. With no clinical acumen, how can they hope to make such judgements? Their *raison d'être* now rests heavily on the possibility of another Dr. Harold Shipman or Lucy Letby occurring.

Regulators completely failed to recognise Dr Shipman and Lucy Letby. With Lucy Letby, they ignored many warnings given to them by senior doctors and nurses.

Medical bureaucrats now have powers to pursue whatever they think is 'in the public interest' (a phrase, lacking specificity, and used to justify their every action). I wonder if they know what, in medical terms, is 'in the public interest', other than avoiding death and irreversible injury. They will claim that their mission to protect the public from doctors and nurses, justifies their means. So who should the public trust more? Would it be their doctor, a politician or a medical practice inspector?

'As bureaucracies accumulate power they become immune to their own mistakes. Instead of changing their stories to fit reality, they can change reality to fit their stories. In the end external reality matches their bureaucratic fantasies, but only because they forced reality to do so.'

Yuval Harari. *'Homo Deus.'* (2015, Random House).

Spiritual

All his life, Sam had been meticulous about running his furniture business, and made sure that everything he did, worked as planned. Then Sam lost his wife. This was because her gynaecologist had overlooked her cervical cancer smear result and failed to review her quickly enough. Sam had a long history of depression, dating back to before he was married. He had undertaken years of medication and psychoanalysis that hardly helped.

Because Sam had remained bereaved for over five years, I gave him a biographical example of another prolonged bereavement. Queen Victoria had remained in a state of mourning for decades after Prince Albert's death, so I recommended he read her biography.

Shortly after, I described Sam's predicament to another patient who I knew to have spiritual leanings. 'Tell him to come to the spiritual church I attend', she said. 'Perhaps someone there might help him'.

Sam was a hard-nosed business owner who believed in nothing he couldn't touch or see, but next time I saw him, I passed on the recommendation. 'What's the catch?' he asked. I told him that there was no cost to it, and that my other patient was sincere when she told me they had helped many. It would seem he had nothing to lose.

One month later Sam returned. He came into my consulting room smiling. 'You will never believe this', he said. He had gone to the church, and was told to take a seat anywhere he liked. He was told to wait until the female medium on the dais, called. 'Is there anyone here called Sam?', she asked.

Sam put his hand in the air, and the medium said, 'I have a message for Sam from a woman known as Letty (a name only he used to call his wife in private; her actual name was Sheila). She says not to continue with such sadness. It's unnecessary. She is happy and says you should get on with your life and be happy too'.

He told me that nobody could have known the special name he used for her. He told me that he knew nobody at the church, and had told nobody he was going. He had no evidence of trickery.

His visit to the church proved transformative. His whole family found the change remarkable. His depression lifted, and he was married eighteen months later. His new wife had known Sheila well, and was happy for him to display her photo in their house, in her memory.

My mother was a spiritual person. Her faith was innocent and untutored, having spent all her early life caring for her older sister. Her sister (the twelfth of thirteen) had been born with Down's Syndrome. She was the daughter of an older mother. Polly died when she was twenty years old, and my mother was heartbroken. Even in her nineties, my mother could still be brought to tears if asked about Polly.

After my father died, I asked her why she seemed not to be too upset. She told me he was with her, always by her side. She would not explain further. 'Some things', she said, 'Words cannot express'.

She was ninety-five-years-old when I visited my mother one afternoon. She said, 'I have something strange to tell you. Yesterday afternoon your father came in and sat down in

his usual chair. Before you say anything, I know he's dead,
but this was so unlike him, never to say a word. I offered
him a cup of tea, but since he didn't respond, I made it
for him, anyway. He left it untouched, got up, and walked
out without saying anything.' She said, 'not saying hello or
goodbye was completely out of character. Being impolite, was
not your father at all!'

The ramblings of a demented old lady, or something
else? She had seen my father as real, and never questioned
the reality of his visit. A few interpretations are possible.

Stalkers

There are patients who will form a personal attachment
to doctors and nurses. They might stalk or harass them.
A witnessed discussion with them is worthwhile trying.
Otherwise, doctors must seek advice from colleagues who
also know the patient. Doctors must consider contacting
their professional indemnity provider and the police.

Stand-ups (No-Shows)

Some patients make appointments, but don't arrive.
Most patients will telephone to cancel; some will not.
No-shows are disruptive and disappointing. Always identify patient unreliability. It sometimes signals disrespect,
but also absent-mindedness or mental illness. Question
the type of doctor-patient relationships you want. In the
small things they do, people show their true nature.

If new patients do not get the appointment they want
(usually asap), they will usually go elsewhere, and not
bother to inform the medical practice. A simple but important lesson to learn in life is that many people say one

thing and mean another. Note who they are. This is most pertinent to dealing with patients from cultures where 'saving face' is critical. They could lose face if they cancel an appointment and have to explain why, so they may choose not to arrive, and not to explain further.

Superman / Superwoman Complex

Many men 'don't do illness'. They think themselves so tough, only a sizeable chunk of Kryptonite would weaken them. They will say, 'Nothing wrong with me, doc! Honestly, I actually don't know why my wife wanted me to come. I'm sorry for wasting your time.'

Some harbour the fantasy that they will live forever or no disease is serious enough to bring them down. Insight may not be one of their strong points. Their outlook could have arisen from fear of a nasty diagnosis, or from the fear a procedure that might hurt them or go wrong. Others never think of illness; their body image is one of unquestioned health.

Getting such patients in touch with their actual state of health can be a challenge. After consulting with them over serious, rather than trivial clinical matters, I would send them a written report. This minimised the possibility of misinterpretation. At least they would have an defined basis for their discussions with friends, relatives and other doctors.

Patience is a virtue when dealing with supermen and women. They may eventually achieve genuine insight and be able to think through their situation. Make your next consultation a combined one; perhaps with a friend or partner who knows them best.

Takers and Users (see Manipulators)

These are people whose desire is to have unpaid servants. Look for the pathognomonic sign: they are demanding from the very start, sometimes even before their first meeting with a doctor.

As I mentioned before under 'Manipulators', many will try to engage a doctor or nurse as their unpaid PA. The commonest request is, 'Could you make an appointment for me' (for testing, or further consultation, etc.). If agreed to, it will involve medical staff making several telephone calls, backwards and forwards. With no access to their diary, it can't be done. Doctors who comply with such demands, will have surrendered to their will. Don't let it happen. Few can afford to play the role of willing servant. If a doctor refuses their requests, they will not get treated graciously.

One rule that applies to all 'takers' is, the more you give, the more they want.

From the darker side of humanity, some have these objectives:

- To gain more and more using any means possible, and

- To gain more while doing less.

Some takers and users are good at hiding. Hidden within many large organisations are those who get paid, regardless of their performance. When pushed to work harder, only the dedicated rise to the challenge; users never feel the need.

Those in receipt of generosity often accuse their donor of meanness, especially if the largesse is reduced or discontinued. Don't be concerned if you are the donor. They will quickly depart for richer pickings, usually without a word of thanks or appreciation.

Paradoxically, those who are rich and more advantaged, are far less likely to show ingratitude. Because the rich get used to attempted rip-offs, they will usually respond gratefully to generosity, and are likely to return favours in one form or another. The under-privileged, who feel they must fight for everything, quickly learn that limited demands are unproductive. As a result they will push all their demands to the limit. They may not understand why so few wish to befriend them.

Many patients are dispassionate users of medical services. All they want is to get 'fixed', and leave. When a doctor retires, or dies, they will not give a second thought to them; they will simply transfer their requests to another convenient provider. This type of patient is completely unfulfilling to deal with. Very little clinical acumen is needed to deal with them. Because developing a doctor-patient relationship is not what they seek, a nurse, paramedic, pharmacist, or a computer avatar will suffice. Because the vast majority of GP consultations are of this type, the large-scale replacement of GPs by alternative health professionals using AI driven computer avatars, is inevitable.

Troublemakers (see Complainers)

There are those who cause trouble wherever they go. They are quick to demand their rights and will try to gain an advantage by listing all the faults they have noticed about a doctor and her practice. Their manner on the telephone, even at first contact, should be a warning of what is to come. Most troublemakers are missing a trick. They will get far more satisfaction if they are respectful, and present a reasonable case. When their approach is aggressive, emotional, dogmatic, incorrect, or unreasonable, they endear no-one.

A lot of troublemakers have failed to receive the respect they think they deserve and so, compensate with aggression. Doctors and nurses who are charitable by nature, might think such people simply misunderstood.

Some savvy troublemakers, know to threaten doctors with GMC notification. They know this will induce fear in most doctors, given the threat to their registration and the years of pointless bureaucratic enquiry that would follow.

In the current climate of litigation, the first thing to do when any verbal dispute arises is to get a witness. The second thing is to verify the complaint. Allow the complainant to speak and repeat back to them what you think they said: 'Now let me see if I heard you correctly. What you want is to sit in our reception area, and eat a meal while waiting to be seen. You would also like your child to run free and have full access to every area of our clinic while you eat. Is that correct?'

Doctors and nurses must make a note of everything that is said and get an independent witness to verify it. Ideally, use CCTV to record every incident. A response to the complainant must follow in writing. Tell them the result of your observations and the thinking behind your assessment and judgement. Follow this with how you intend to resolve the issue. The case alluded to before, involved a patient (not one of mine) eating a curry in my practice waiting area. It would have been better had we placed a large notice banning eating, and restricting public entry to all staff areas, but we had never needed to do so before.

In my clinic, we never encouraged the return of patients behaving unacceptably (making my staff and others feel uncomfortable). There are plenty of other doctors for such people to aggravate.

Type A & B

What makes a Type 'A' person? Friedman and Rosenman (1970s), two Californian cardiologists, developed the theory of 'time urgency'. Type A behaviour may be 'natural' to some, but it can also develop temporarily in those experiencing time restriction.

Type 'B' characters typically plan everything they do and act at leisure. They take their time, rarely hurry, and allow plenty of redundancy in their time schedule. The plan is to have time to spare and to avoid being rushed.

Jimmy had to catch a flight at mid-day. He awoke at 5am and went to his office first. He had letters to dictate and some business matters to sort out. It was his mother's birthday, so he wanted to buy her some flowers on the way to the airport. He planned to visit her briefly, then get on his way. His wife had sent a message to warn him not to forget his daughter's birthday.

He arrived at the airport with only 20 minutes to spare. He checked-in, and had only just cleared security when he heard his name being called. They were about to close the gate as he arrived panting, after running to get there on time. A Type 'A' character, Jim exhibited this behaviour as a feature of his badly planned, overburdened lifestyle (all of his own making).

Coronary atheroma (artery 'furring') always precedes cardiac infarction, with very few exceptions. Without atheroma, Type 'A' behaviour is unlikely to cause cardiac infarction. For those with critical coronary artery stenoses, Type 'A' more than Type 'B' behaviour, will reduce exercise tolerance and increase the risk of a coronary occlusion. Friedman and Rosenman showed that those with Type 'A' Behaviour, have double the cardiac infarction risk of those who are Type B.

Vanities and Gods

Human vanity has psychological consequences, and some doctors will be called upon to deal with them. The consequences are not all harmless.

With the latest media services at our fingertips, we can now peer into the lives of others and compare 'them' to 'us'. If the Buddha was correct, and the chief cause of psychological stress is avarice, collecting admirable possessions to distinguish ourselves has always been a common mission. Now that social media allows others to view our possessions, the opportunities for avarice have multiplied. Comparing possessions and relationships on-line has led to a new form of stress - cyber-bullying.

Greek mythology makes obvious the profound differences between the gods and mere mortals. Many of us now harbour the fantasy that we, too, should have god-like attributes. The promises made in cosmetic and exercise-related adverts, continue to suggest we can get close to them. Some humans now feel they already share some of the mythical strength, some of the beauty, and some of the wisdom of the gods. Many now fantasise about eternal youth, and spend a fortune trying to achieve it. As our quality of life improves, the more attractive immortality becomes (at least for those still fertile and full of hope). Unfortunately, only mythical creatures are immortal and able to perform miraculous deeds.

Those who have marketed medical interventions over the millennia, have made a lot of promises to the middle-aged. Some are that cosmetics will keep their skin youthful and exercise will extend their youth as well as giving them six-pack 'abs' (abdominal muscles). The object is to attract more admirers.

I have known vitamin and mineral supplement manufacturers to promise the avoidance of hair loss, the maintenance of vision in old age, and enough libidinous energy to conserve youthful sexuality. Unfortunately, there are just as many promises made by medical science. One is that a cure for cancer and heart disease will be here soon, as long as we spend enough money on research. One genetically engineered step further, and we might all join the gods in having eternal life. Look what humanity has achieved since 1900, so just imagine what the next hundred years will bring. (This is inductive reasoning. At best, it is no bad thing to support hope, promise, and expectation).

The young only rarely need to consider their mortality, and seldom feel any different from the Gods (now called super heroes).

One hundred and fifty years ago, patients would have been more in touch with illness and death. Many lived in overcrowded, deprived conditions, and many died young from infectious diseases. Pneumonia and streptococcal throat infections spread easily. Diphtheria and TB were common. The resulting funerals of children were frequent, and the average life expectancy was 40-years. Now perfect health and improved longevity are what many seek. After all, adverts continually remind us all that *'we are worth it.'*

There are millions of people driven by vanity; many spending fortunes on chasing or reclaiming their youth. Luckily for them, an army of (medical) 'professionals' lies in wait, ready and willing to encourage any of their delusions. Growth hormone, B12 and anabolic steroid injections, personal gym-training, dietary advice, and multi-factor food supplementation, all claim to provide an elixir.

There is nothing much wrong with trying to preserve youth as age progresses, but for doctors focused on illness, pandering to the vain gets tiresome by comparison. The vain are much less tiresome when they have some insight into the current biological limitations of retaining youth. Some caution is required because genetic engineering is fast gaining the potential to change what was once impossible. Transforming chromosome telomere nucleotide chemistry may eventually improve longevity in humans.

At the moment, we cannot stop the appearances of aging for long. In the short term, however, I have seen faces made to look 10-years younger, after the removal of pendulous eyelids and sagging neck folds. I have also seen aesthetic horrors: tightly stretched, wind-blasted faces resulting from face-lifts. I have also seen unnaturally large and rigid breast implants, completely out of proportion to the patient's body size. Democracy and capitalism have worked to foster freedom of choice, and enough freedom to indulge in as much delusion as we can afford.

There is no need to denigrate the vain and the vacuous; they do that well enough for themselves. While a few doctors specialise in serving the needs of the vain, others believe there is no place for it. For those cosmetic surgeons engaged in serious reconstructive work, a side-line of vanity work will provide them with a steady private income.

Some of the 'perfect' health features now sought are:

- Voluptuous breasts (Jane Russell, and Marilyn Monroe – showing my age) - not now required for fame. Julia Roberts, in the 1999 film *'Notting Hill'* (PolyGram Filmed Entertainment) rhetorically questioned their attraction to men. Her comment: *'Men and nudity. Huh! Particularly breasts . . . they're just breasts. Every second person has them!'*

- Pouting, oversized 'fish' lips (comparable to the Giant Grouper).

- An enviable body weight and shape equal to any bulimic / anorexic fashion model.(see my book 'Who Loses Wins' (2024);

- A six-pack abdomen, and compact 'butt'.

- Sufficient height to attract beautiful creatures. Although Danny DeVito is only 4 feet, 9 and 3/4 inches tall, he has many admirers.

- Dainty feet (Judy Garland, and Cinderella);

- A complete absence of grey hair and wrinkles.

- A beautiful coiffure, or depilation: pubic, cephalic and axillary (varies with country and culture).

- A breath-taking penis size, or tidy labia.

- Floral scented armpits (*de rigueur* everywhere, except on building sites).

The vain will ignore sensible advice if it doesn't suit their purpose. Most can hear, but few will listen and learn. Appealing adverts can suffer a similar fate; we might enjoy the advert but not remember the product.

Instead of vain aspirations, improved health and disease prevention should be more desirable. One problem is that doctors too often offer clichés for advice. These can bore patients rather than help to change their minds. Although true, some yawn-inducing examples are:

- Don't smoke.

- Don't drink too much alcohol.

- Don't overexpose yourself to sunlight without protection.

- Eat less. Exercise more. Get fit. Keep fit (preferably to an athletic standard).

- Eat healthily (well established scientifically, but often based on the prevailing, ever-changing fashion). You can read my books: *'Eat to Your Heart's Content',* and *'Heart Sense',* to find out which foods contain the nutrients which might, in theory, reduce arterial atherogenesis (the process of artery 'furring') - a major cause of middle-age mortality.

Some advice is correct, but unrealistic. Why advocate smoking cessation to those over 70-years-old (assuming they smoke in isolation), or suggest the poor eat five pieces of fruit or vegetables every day, when some fruit is expensive (a remark made by Prof. Helen Stokes-Lampard, Chair, RCGP Council).

During the North African desert campaign of World War 2, Winston Churchill visited Field Marshall Montgomery ('Monty') in his caravan. They ate a meagre lunch. Monty announced: 'I neither smoke nor drink alcohol, and I am 100% fit'. Churchill, the epicurean, replied: 'I drink and smoke, and I am 200% fit.'

Churchill lived for ninety years, and 'Monty' for eighty-eight. Although Churchill suffered a few cardiac and cerebral infarcts, I very much doubt he regretted smoking cigars, or one morsel of his gourmet diet. Genetic profile, not food, controls longevity most. Because this is an unpopular idea, the media will usually edit it out.

Vulnerable Patients

This subject needs its own treatise. Older adults, children, the demented and the confused, are all vulnerable to the adverse will of others.

Without sufficient life experience, and having not reached the age of consent, some children are at risk from the adults in charge of their care. We need a greater awareness of the welfare of young carers, those performing poorly at school, slow developers and parents who are uncompromising with their children.

Abuse comes in many forms; some obvious, some not. Among them are physical abuse (look-out for unexplained bruises and injuries); emotional abuse (bullying, threatening, ridiculing, disrespectful, and demeaning behaviour); neglect; sexual abuse, and financial or institutional abuse. Love, embarrassment, and the fear of reprisal will stop some adults reporting abuse. As in all human affairs, there are strong associations with poverty and wealth, socio-economic class, and educational attainment.

The Wealthy

Is 'old money' more acceptable than 'new money'? Money was once a taboo subject for the rich and privileged. After all, when money is taken for granted, what is there to discuss? Many once deemed the discussion of money vulgar, especially if it was made from slavery, child labour or criminal activity.

Those with 'new money' are much more likely to flaunt it, especially if they came from poverty. I have known them say, *'I want the best, and I don't care how much it costs'.* That is usually before they know the cost. They are likely to be impressed by the trappings of a doctor's success – a fashionable address, smart consulting room décor and state-of-the-art equipment. The alpha-male behaviour of some doctors who distance themselves from patients, with large intervening desks and dutiful, uniformed staff in attendance, will impress them. Unfortunately for the profligate, none of these are reliable enough indicators of a doctor's expertise.

Those who have built their own businesses will have used tight expenditure control to create their wealth. Thrift, not largesse or fantasy, has more often led to their businesses becoming successful. Some wealthy business people will try to exert the same control over their clinical management as private patients. I welcomed it when it favoured sensible compliance, but not when it created demands for irrelevant tests and interventions. Those who had come to trust me were usually quick to recognise clinical reality. Some very rich people, having achieved much success in life, may come to believe in their infallibility.

I had a billionaire patient with blackouts who refused for over one year to have a much needed pacemaker implanted. Was his resistance to the procedure motivated by the cost, the inconvenience, or by ignorance and fear of the procedure and its benefits? After a pacemaker implantation, he had no further blackouts. I resisted saying, 'I told you so!'

Two advantages of practicing privately are continuity and more predictable patient compliance. With no time restrictions, and time for full discussion, patients can gain a full understanding of their condition. The quick return of their laboratory results, and the absence of any waiting list, were other advantages. These factors all benefit clinical outcome.

A simple, but shocking fact, is that far fewer private than NHS patients die on waiting lists or go blind because of untreated glaucoma. The question is, what part has government interference and UK medical bureaucracy, played in the growing divide, especially now that doctors are no longer executive controllers of medical practice. Before we accept political control further, should we not know the answer to one question? What contribution have medical bureaucrats made to patient morbidity and mortality? A full public enquiry is appropriate, because my guess is that they have increased both, and now waste public money. I would suggest that regulators and NHS executives are not acting solely 'in the public interest'.

Wealth allows the rich to demand 'the best', and ask for 'the best that money can buy'. This has sometimes resulted in my patients travelling to other countries for treatment. Despite what advocates of the NHS believe, the UK is not the only place where world-class medical expertise can be found. Wealth allows unrestricted choice, and a wider range of medical possibilities, but accusations of élitism rarely concern those whose lives are at stake.

Art thou poor, yet hast thou golden slumbers?
O sweet content.
Art thou rich, yet is thy mind perplex'd?
O punishment.

'Sweet Content.'
Thomas Dekker (1575 – 1641).

Wimps?

Also known as '(snow) flakes', those who dither and constantly change their mind, can also be afraid of their own shadow. Some people just can't take the physical, emotional, or cognitive demands of life, and they must choose their lifestyle carefully. People dither for other reasons. Some are in distress. Some are so pre-occupied with personal problems they could drive their vehicle into a brick wall. The resulting injuries, should they survive them, could put them into hospital. It seems harsh to mention it, but some patients find their illness or injury a convenience. It can give them time to consider their life and how to cope with it. Hospital admission will remove them from the tribulations of life and allow them to think.

A sympathetic clinical approach from doctors and nurses is appropriate. Some who feel stressed by their life will have hypertension, increased blood coagulability, reduced immune resistance, inappropriate changes in behaviour and depression. When pushed towards a metaphorical medical cliff-edge, one further stress could bring about a sudden dramatic change; perhaps a catastrophic medical event. In the tough days following the 2nd World War, fractures and serious medical conditions were the only medical conditions seen as legitimate. The results of stress and deteriorating mental health remained unacceptable excuses for poor functioning.

To get the full psychosocial-behavioural picture of such patients, a conversation with their parents, partner, friends, or work-mates will often be necessary. Doctors versed in the art of medicine will know this; those who are not, should limit themselves to fracture management.

WISC: Wolf In Sheep's Clothing

These patients may act as if they are innocent and naïve, but they are smart and manipulative. Some patients will use this ploy to get what they want from doctors. Their assumption is that doctors won't see through their artifice. Given that few doctors are as street-wise as their patients, they could be right.

CHAPTER THREE

HOW DOCTORS AND NURSES MANAGE PATIENTS, AND HOW PATIENTS MANAGE TO SURVIVE

Patients do not want to be treated as numbers (the patient in bed 15), or diseases (the patient with MS), but as individual sentient beings.

Many patients need help to help themselves.

Patients should choose doctors whose source of gratification and self-esteem comes from improving their patients' physical and mental state.

Communication between patients and doctors is at its best when all differences in culture, intelligence, knowledge and behaviour are resolved by respect and understanding.

Clinical judgements, and the giving of pertinent advice, are both essential clinical arts. Understanding disease is merely a matter of science.

I have made an important assumption in this chapter: that the patients referred to are conscious, and able to communicate without cognitive impairment. I have not addressed the considerable problems associated with safe-guarding those with reduced mental capacity, and those who are unconscious for whatever reason.

The patients a doctor, nurse, pharmacist, physiother-apist, osteopath or paramedic will meet will form a group that overlaps those described before under 'Doc-tors and Nurses as Characters'.

Doctors, nurses, patients, administrators and regula-tors, all populate the same human jungle, and failure to understand the creatures living there can have serious consequences.

We will all have met some notable characters at school, but as a nurse or doctor, we will meet those we don't identify with. Our colleagues are in part pre-se-lected by social background and education, but pa-tients and our relationships with them are another mat-ter. How doctors and nurses relate to patients is the subject of this chapter.

It has always been a challenge to discover the true nature of our fellow beings, and to see passed the image they choose to portray. In the past, gaining insight into the character of a colleague was a relatively easy matter because they mostly came from the same social background. To-day, medical students and patients in the UK come from more diverse social backgrounds. Gaining insight into patients and colleagues with their greater diversity is now more difficult.

By choosing to distance themselves from gaining insight into their patients and their circumstances, some doctors will become less effective clinically. We make the best clinical judgements when using a complete clinical picture together with all the pertinent meta-data about each patient, the most telling of which will be visible to any fly-on-the-wall. The further away one gets from the reality of what our patients experience, the less reliable will be our judgments of them. Exposure, limited to the medical facts alone, is a risk to patient management. To practise medicine effectively often requires time spent getting to know each patient. In the NHS, however, the need for improved corporate efficiency has led to consultation times being shortened. Patient through-put and efficient handling are the measures now sought, even though they can diminish the application of clinical judgement, medical wisdom and an improved quality of care for patients.

That reduced patient morbidity and mortality are the primary aims of medical practice, needs to be remembered at all times. If medical executives are achieving neither, we must question their existence.

Some wealthy nations have gone further than the relief of symptoms; they have invested in prevention and the early detection of disease. The statement *prevention is better than cure* may be a worn-out cliché, but it is one dear to patients. Patients rather than some doctors, also see the sense in making diagnoses as early as possible, while for many decades the NHS focussed only on overt disease. Over the last five decades, UK doctors have slowly accepted prevention as a new role. When I first offered medical screening to my patients in 1973 (for early detection and prevention), my colleagues thought it a waste of time, and merely a money making exercise.

Helping patients to overcome their symptoms is a major source of self-esteem for doctors and nurses. For all doctors, the satisfaction derived from helping patients is enough reason for them to continue work. For a few, there is another, old-fashioned longer-term benefit: the accumulation of patients who become trusted patients, friends and supporters. All jobs done well can provide a sense of worth, but not much can compare with taking responsibility for patients and helping them to live healthily. This is altruism, not self-indulgence at work. Apart from doctors, nurses, and paramedics, everyone with patient contact can share in this, whether they be floor cleaners, porters, or those who serve food to patients. Few medical professionals have difficulty justifying their existence, with some gaining even further satisfaction from taking part in an effective specialised team.

Desirable Patients?

The best of personal relationships require no effort.

A few patient characteristics influence the doctor-patient relationship. Foremost among them is educational attainment. Patients vary a lot in the vocabulary and language skills they bring to describing their problems. Age, gender, socio-economic class and culture also exert an influence. Coincidentally, these also determine longevity and morbidity.

The form each consultation takes can depend on location. I found quite a difference (in the 1970s) between those patients who attended St. George's Hospital at Hyde Park Corner, London SW1, and those who came to St. George's Hospital Tooting, in South London. The inhabitants of these areas have changed in the last 55 years, but distinct contrasts remain. Some doctors and nurses might prefer a particular patient demographic, and they should give due consideration to where they choose to work. Demography is a major factor in determining clinical outcomes.

Gender not only determines the prevalence of some diseases, but also the nature of the doctor-patient relationship. One can assume (until proven otherwise) for instance, that female patients (those with 'XX' chromosomes) are more open communicators; more in touch with their emotions, and braver in medical matters than men. Even when afraid, women more than men will readily agree to necessary medical interventions.

Age has many and various effects on the doctor-patient relationship. There is no reliable relationship between age and wisdom, but with age, outspokenness often becomes evident. At my age, I have nothing to lose by expressing my opinions; I am not looking for a job, and I have no duty to please others. When dealing with the retired, prepare for comments prefaced by 'When I was a young . . .' or 'Back in the day . . .' What will follow might be of interest, but may lack current relevance. Because many trends get recycled, the outspokenness of age is sometimes worth listening to.

There is much to understand about the differing attitudes expressed by the rich and the poor. They are different enough in my experience to regard them a separate cultures. Since cancer and heart disease rates are three to five times greater in the poor, this subject is a vital one.

Which aspects of a patient's individual personality bring most joy or dismay to those caring for them? For me, it was always the interesting, charming, appreciative, experienced, passionate and intelligent patients who brought me the most joy. It was how demanding, devious, arrogant, or obsessional patients were that brought me most dismay. It mattered whether patients were users, abusers, or seducers, and whether they were honest professionals or dishonest scoundrels. Like all others, doctors and nurses will have a list of characters they like and dislike. Although trained medical professionals will not voice such views, they can affect the doctor-patient relationship.

No doctor or nurse can choose their patients directly, so any question of who might be best is rhetorical. Our calling is to serve all who suffer.

I was once told by a shipping billionaire what talent had helped him most in business. It was his talent for choosing people (implying an ability to understand others).

Mrs. Anita Griggs, Head of Falkner House School, London, can choose those 5-year-old girls, likely to excel as educated, successful women, whatever path they choose to follow in life. For many decades, the reputation of her school has depended on her ability to judge the potential of young children. She once referred to it as 'a black art'.

The art of understanding others is basic to practising the art of medicine.

In all fields of human endeavour, it is easier to deal with friendly, helpful people. If they are well-informed, intelligent, perceptive, and have insight, so much the better. As far as patients are concerned, it helps if they are willing and

DOCTORS, NURSES AND PATIENTS 175

able to learn, and can accept critical discussion. Successful medical management depends on patient compliance, and that will usually (but not always) follow once patients understanding their medical issues.

Some do not need to understand; they already trust doctors and nurses enough, coming as they do with a readymade faith in the judgement of medical professionals. When I first started in medical practice, this was how it was; trust accepted without question. Now they have powers well beyond their capability, many administrators and regulators with little respect for doctors or nurses, squirm at the thought.

What Do Patients Need to Know?

All patients should consider this question: how can I get enough personal consideration from the doctors and nurses dealing with me? We all have preferences for how we wish to be treated by others, so here are a few things patients need to know.

Because it makes light work of every consultation, most doctors prefer pleasant, intelligent patients, capable of giving a focused account of their symptoms and observations, rather than descriptions that date from 'once upon a time'. My preference was for patients who welcomed time spent on discussion, whether it be their history, my assessments, diagnoses, suggested investigations, or my proposed management strategy. Patients who need quick-fixes will do just as well with a nurse practitioner, physician associate or pharmacist, rather than a doctor. In my practice, I mostly dealt with complicated cases; those who other doctors failed to diagnose or help. To solve their more complicated problems required two key elements:

• Detailed knowledge of the patient and their pertaining circumstances, and

• Time for in-depth discussion.

Most patients are a pleasure to meet. Very few will cause a feeling of heart-sink and be tiresome to deal with. I met only two such patients in fifty-three years of practice. As a matter of duty, we have to deal with all-comers, but the more reasonable and polite the patient, the more a doctor or nurse will warm to them and want to help. Those patients who are consistently unpleasant (as when demanding their rights as a citizen), will be lucky to establish a mutually rewarding doctor-patient relationship. It would be better for them to find a more compatible doctor. A surprise may await them. They may end up with a doctor who is even less tolerant of their discordant behaviour. Since doctors get the patients they deserve, and patients get the doctors they deserve, so some patient redistribution is inevitable.

Some patients change their outlook and attitude daily, depending on their pain, anxiety, fear, suffering and contentment at the time of consultation. In the following summary, I have listed my preferences (in no particular order) for those patient characteristics which promote a pleasant and successful doctor-patient relationship. Such patients are:

1. Succinct, objective historians.

2. Honest and dependable.

3. Respectful.

4. Intelligent, logical, and educated.

5. Modest.

6. Pleasant, and sensitive to others.

7. Humorous.

8. Coordinated, with efficient executive functionality.

9. Relaxed.

10. Not overly obsessive.

Mutual compatibility is the key. It defines the nature, progress, and prognosis of every doctor
patient relationship.

Full of what seemed to be ridiculous, unshakable ideas, Ms. S. G. was getting worse day by day. Her local NHS hospital had failed to diagnose her. She was, however, too angry and insufficiently literate to recount her history meaningfully. She didn't want discussion; she wanted action. In desperation, she demanded admission to hospital. She had felt so ill since giving birth to her son a few months earlier, she now felt the need for something to be done fast. The diagnosis was fairly obvious. I diagnosed Sheehan's syndrome: postpartum pituitary / adrenal malfunction. Paraphrasing Spike Milligan's epitaph: she knew she was ill.

Her clinical situation was urgent (she was hypotensive, and hyponatraemic), so was her medico-legal situation. Out of

desperation, she was ready to accuse everyone of incompe-
tence. Since nobody had diagnosed her condition correctly,
many of her accusations of incompetence were well-founded.
As it so often is, the main diagnostic clue was in her history;
only later was the diagnosis verified by the investigations.
Following the correct diagnosis and the correct hormone re-
placement, she made a rapid recovery.

Ms. S. G. was too sick to display any of the most helpful patient characteristics. Once she recovered though, she
displayed them all.

Beware: it is difficult to see the truth about a person
and their clinical situation when they present in a cloud of
frustration and anger and are making illogical demands. Effective clinical practice (that which satisfies all concerned)
will often depend on our understanding of patients and
their understanding of us. In particular, they need to know
that we are knowledgeable enough, and able enough, to
make happen what needs to happen.

It Takes all Sorts

'Men go to gape at mountain peaks, at the boundless tides
of the sea, the broad sweep of the rivers, the encircling ocean
and the motions of the stars: and yet they leave themselves
unnoticed; they do not marvel at themselves.'

St. Augustine:
'Confessions.'

From a doctor's point of view, there are several ways to
classify patients, none of which are worthwhile unless they
help us to manage patients better. It is not a doctor's brief
to sit in judgement on patients, but it would be naïve to
ignore a patient's psychological and personality attributes

and the influence they can have. The challenge is to deal with all-comers, and to benefit as many patients as possible.

We all have personality and behavioural characteristics that vary as any spectrum does between extremes. The face we present will vary between these extremes and change from time to time. Here are some of the relevant outlook continua that apply to patients, nurses and doctors:

Academic – Non-academic
Aggressive / combative – Placid/ non-combative.
Arrogant – Humble
Attached - Detached
Balanced views – Polarised views.
Bi-(multi)lingual – Native tongue only.
Charming – Uncouth.
Courageous – Easily frightened

Communicative – Non-communicative.
Co-operative – Non-co-operative.
Cranky ideas – Well-founded ideas
Eager to say either : 'I know my rights' - or 'I know my duties.'
Educated – Uneducated
Egoist – Reserved
Empathetic – Apathetic
Extravert – Introvert
Focussed - Unfocussed.
Friendly – Unfriendly.
Honest – Dishonest.
Humorous – Humourless.
Ignorant - Knowledgeable
Intelligent - Unintelligent.
Literate – Illiterate

Low - High Socio-Economic class.
Numerate – Enumerate
Objective – Non-objective
Obsequious – Challenging
Obsessional - Easy-going
Opinionated – Open-minded
Professional – Unprofessional.
Sympathetic – Unsympathetic
Threatening – Supportive
Vain - Modest
Worldly wise – Closeted.

And for those with psychiatric states:

Deluded / Hallucinatory – Sane.
Depressed / Withdrawn – Happy / Open.
Fearful – Brave.
Relaxed – Anxious.

For those with drug states (alcohol and drugs of abuse)

Dangerous – Harmless.
Deluded / Hallucinatory – Well oriented.
Under the influence of drugs – Sober.
Uncontrolled – In control.
Violent – Non-violent,
etc.

Despite the artificial nature of this list, and the considerable overlap between the entities, it is easily possible for each of us to choose which type of person we prefer to deal with. This will be relevant for patients only when they are free to choose their doctor (except for private patients, this mostly exists only outside of the UK).

One of the most charming and valued, long-standing patients of mine was Joe Satchell. I attended his funeral in September 2016. I wanted to pay tribute to him here. As a measure of the man, Joe would send flowers to my receptionists for no reason other than he had cancelled an appointment. In this, he was unique among my 20,000 patients. We missed his presence as a cultured, affable patient and friend.

Contrast Joe, with those who try to claim compensation against doctors and nurses, on what may seem like unreasonable grounds. It became more easily possible after the introduction of *pro bono,* 'no win, no fee' legal arrangements. The NHS receives 10,000 claims for compensation each year, and recently faced paying £4.3 billion in compensation. Many of these claims for medical negligence are substantiated. Some have made a small fortune, given that almost anyone aggrieved can now bring a negligence claim.

Every disease has its risks, as does every medical practice intervention. Doctors and nurses have to resign themselves to being easy targets, given the mishaps that are bound to occur when performing the inherently risky work of investigating and treating patients. No intervention, including a consultation, is without risk. In the utopian view held by many medical administrators and regulators, most of whom have never practiced medicine (and even some who have), medical practice should be risk free. The utopian world they seek may exist, but not on this planet.

In the 1970s, Ivan Illich noted that litigation has made even first-aiders think twice before becoming a Good Samaritan.

Medical regulators claim that their work reduces the risks patients suffer at the hands of doctors and nurses. It is not their brief to acknowledge the risks intrinsic to all human activity. They are always ready to accuse doctors of exposing patients to unnecessary risk, even if they have never managed patient risk, or experienced clinical work themselves. Their statutory power allows them to punish medical professionals for what they see as not being 'in the public interest'. The idea on which this is based is metaphysical: that every citizen deserves the right to live in a world free of risk.

Although no doctor can choose their patients direct-ly, private patients can choose their doctor and hospital (while rare in the NHS, it is usual throughout the rest of the world). Although patients may be given the choice of a GP in primary care NHS practices, that rarely guarantees which doctor they will see. In private practice, patients can choose who they consult, and can change without retribution.

Patient choice should be based on medical reputation, but is more often based on availability. Hopefully, any reputation a doctor has will be based on her knowledge, experience, and ability to deal successfully with medical problems. It is more likely, however, that affability will bring the most favour. Once a patient has developed a worthwhile rapport with a doctor, availability becomes a lesser issue.

For a clinical management plan to work well, the advan-tage lies with patients who understand their condition, the time-scale involved, and the objectives of any treatment.

From a patient's perspective, the acceptability of the doctor-patient relationship is all important. How are pa-tients to know that the only reliable measures of a doctor's ability rest on their diagnostic proficiency, their case management ability, and the improvements they can make to patient morbidity and mortality?

Nobody can satisfy every patient, but our duty is to try. Try as we might, there will always be some we cannot help, sometimes because of personal incompatibility. In 53-years, I encountered only six such patients. I thought it better to refer them to other doctors. There must have been many others who, having sensed our mutual incompatibility, chose never to return.

The threshold to doctor-patient incompatibility has changed in recent decades. The trend is now for patients to consult 'Doctor Google', and to think they know best, even when they have no medical knowledge, technical know-how, medical experience or clinical perspective. This trend has gained momentum as younger patients have replaced older ones. It parallels the growing obligation to accept social equality while forsaking educational inequality. That everyone has a valid view has fast become acceptable. Antipathy towards expertise and science has accompanied it. Social media has given both the informed and ill-informed an equal voice, and the doctor-patient relationship must accommodate to the change.

Patient Scenarios

'All the world's a stage . . .'

As You Like It. Act 2, Scene 7. William Shakespeare.

On every stage, the actors and the scenery together can make a play come alive. Regardless of our character, we must all function on a stage playing out our own life scenario. We can accept our scenario as unavoidable, or one to be chosen in every detail. Whether at home or at work, some scenarios can either trigger the onset of a disease or modify its progress. To consider the relevance of this, all we have to do is compare a typical wealthy scenario with one of deprivation: a five-fold difference in cancer and cardiovascular disease prevalence results in a social health divide.

Although we have yet to define all the genotypic details of every individual, we cannot ignore unhealthy scenarios and their aetiological significance. To understand and find the relevance to patients of different scenarios is to practise the art of medicine. From experience, I have often found that understanding these considerations gave me a clinical advantage. Many patients will respect those doctors and nurses who take an interest in their circumstances. Many believe that their medical problems arise there, but know that too few doctors are interested. Other patients will see no connection between the two, and must have to have it pointed out to them.

Many patients conflate health and disease. Although they are separate entities, disease can affect health, and diminished health can affect disease processes (depression can enhance cancer progression, for instance). Diet can affect health, but is of doubtful relevance to the origin of the most common 'killer' diseases (cancer and artery 'furring' or atherosclerosis).

Some theories of aetiology are controversial. For instance, can one cigarette induce lung cancer? Can one virus infection initiate a chronic auto-immune disease? Time-links affect causes and susceptibility. Men do not go bald aged thirteen, but many will see some hair loss after 20-years of age. Acne appears at puberty, not usually before. Some women become hypertensive only as their menopause progresses.

Love Lost and Lonely

Joe was a 65-year-old widower. He had everything he wanted in life, except a partner. His wife had died from leukaemia some years before. His regular gardener had fallen ill and a woman, forty years his junior, had replaced him. They fell in love at first sight; not something either expected to happen.

He had sought my clinical advice for many decades, and so we had a close doctor-patient relationship. His last consultation concerned his angina. This time, he wanted my pastoral advice, given all I knew all about his personal circumstances and medical condition. His question was: 'What should I do about this unexpected new relationship?' I replied with a rhetorical question: 'What have you got to lose?' This agreed with his own view of the relationship. Not only had it relieved his bereavement and loneliness, it had unexpectedly improved his angina.

Following a coronary bypass (CABG) many years before, we failed to place a stent in one of Joe's extensively narrowed arteries (his distal anterior descending coronary artery). I told him then we could do no more for him. It was a surprise to observe, therefore, how his new relationship had improved his exercise performance.

Joe's arteries could not have changed much over the short course of his new relationship, so how might one explain his improvement? Could it be that happiness had raised his exercise threshold to angina (by reducing his catecholamine drive and myocardial oxygen demand)? It is certainly worthy of further research. It is interesting to note that Heberden's original description (in 1768) of chest tightness (angina) included emotion as a provocative factor.

There is another historical snippet of cardiovascular research that brings emotion and the heart together. William Harvey's book, made him famous by describing the circulation of blood (*de Motu Cordis*, 1628). Harvey, however, was concerned as much with how human emotion affects the pulse rate, as he was with the circulation of the blood. After all his research, he could find no connection. That is because the autonomic nervous system connecting the brain to the heart had yet to be discovered. That had to wait until the 19th century, and the work of many, including Claude Bernard, A.V. Waller, the Weber brothers. It was J.N. Langley FRS, who coined the phrase 'autonomic nervous system' (Langley J. Observations on the physiological action of extracts of the supra-renal bodies. J. Physiology. 1901; 27:237-256).

If physicians delegate all consideration of their patient's emotional state to psychologists, psychiatrists, and counsellors (bureaucratic rules to be followed concerning referral to certificated experts), it could lead to clinical mistakes. A collegiate, interdisciplinary approach, however, usually works well for patients. Here is an unusual example of the collegiate approach in action.

Mr. B. was wealthy enough to own his own small island in the Caribbean. Twenty years before I came to know him, he developed prostate cancer, but was now responding poorly

to treatment. He organised and paid for an annual inter-
national conference to discuss the subject. He invited many
specialists to enjoy a brief holiday on his exotic island. His
only request was that they reviewed his case management for
one whole session of the conference.

Pre-patients?

Not all patients with diseases have symptoms. This presents a problem for doctors trying to make early diagnoses.
With no prognostic advantage, early diagnosis can be irrelevant. This will apply to some cancers, to some neu-
rodegenerative diseases like multiple sclerosis and motor
neurone disease, and to many other conditions for which
there is no cure. At least early diagnosis will allow early
management plans to be made.

There are many early diagnoses that can lead to an improved prognosis. Take as an example, the early detection
of atheromatous disease (artery 'furring'), using harmless
carotid arterial ultrasound screening. A simple screening
test detects the disease process responsible for almost 50%
of middle-aged deaths in the western world. Using this
technique, one can detect atherosclerosis decades before it
causes symptoms, and well before any sign of a coronary
or cerebral problem (using exercise ECG, a stress echocar-
diogram, or perfusion study). 'Statin' drugs, given early
enough, can reduce or stop its progress , and will significantly reduce the risk of heart attacks and some strokes.

Some investigations return results that are only a little more predictive than tossing a coin. Abnormal blood
lipids levels are factors used in the cardiovascular risk
calculation, 'qRisk3'. Although of epidemiological value,
qrisk3 will detect only 60% of individuals with carotid

atheroma. Tossing a coin correctly predicts it in 50% of them!

The treatment and life-style changes motivated by the early detection of a potentially fatal disease like atherosclerosis have the potential to reduce morbidity and mortality. Proof of a population benefit, however, is required before being funded with public money. My private patients had a head-start; I prescribed a 'statin' (HMG-CoA Reductase Inhibitor) to all those with proven atheroma (the cause of most cardiovascular risk), even if they had 'normal' blood lipids, and especially if they had a positive family history and a low HDL cholesterol component.

Because neither biological clocks, nor atheroma can be reversed, my patients accepted that a 20-year advantage would be worth paying for (given the small relative cost of an ultrasound test). The only downside was the treatment. Statin drugs have side-effects (in up to 50% of patients). The early discovery of atheroma had other worthwhile benefits. It motivated weight reduction, dietary improvement, and improved physical fitness.

Those antipathetic to screening are right to be concerned about inducing anxiety and turning healthy people into patients. I saw this quite infrequently. Screening more often re-assures, simply because the commonest outcome of screening is to find nothing of clinical interest.

Doctors and public health authorities try not to scare the public. The media more often spread fear and panic, not always justifiably. As the coronavirus progressed across the world (from March 2020), one newspaper suggested that we were all about to face a 'killer' virus. That led to many patients with pre-existing respiratory and other serious con-

ditions to self-isolate. They retreated to their bunkers, fully stocked with food and toilet rolls (the panic-buying of which reduced wholesale stocks in the UK for some time).

Although there has been some shift in opinion in the last 50-years about the value of screening (NHS GPs earn a fee-for-service for simple screening), the prevailing medical culture (the standard medical model) remains as it should, centred on the diagnosis and treatment of symptomatic disease. Since many doctors are at their happiest making 'interesting' diagnoses (according to Ivan Illich), they are not much enthused by what they take to be pointless medical screening. The benefits of routine mammography, cervical smears, PSA testing, BP evaluation, and diabetic checks, however, are undeniable.

The finding of pre-symptomatic early cases usually counters any negative attitudes towards screening, although by definition, the process is only worthwhile once an improvement in clinical outcome has been shown. As a matter of personal outlook, there remains a divide between doctors who want to 'put out fires', and those who want to 'prevent fires'. Since they are not mutually exclusive, why not master both? My long exposure to the consequences of disease motivated me to want to prevent it, but other doctors have a different perspective.

The ongoing discussion in the public sector relates to the cost effectiveness of preventative medicine. This has never applied to the private sector, where patients get screened for common sense reasons, with no need for the financial justifications of the public sector. It is understandable that those who might spend public money on screening, must first confirm sufficient diagnostic accuracy and the prognostic value of the interventions proposed.

My private patients decided 50-years ago that screening was sensible and were happy to pay for the assessment, the reassurance and the navigational advice it provides. The diagnostic accuracy on which such advice is based is an important issue all pre-patients should know. Technology easily fools patients, especially with the use of smart new, state-of-the-art equipment. They will rarely question its accuracy or dependability, but continue to believe that screening procedures are a wise precaution.

There are some practical problems with prevention. Too few people (potential patients) tempt providence by asking: *'is there something wrong with me that would be better managed earlier rather than later?'* In my practice, many came for cardiac screening because a friend or relative had died unexpectedly. We often saw the wrong people (those who were anxious, and low risk); obviously, someone should have made an earlier assessment of the friend or relative who died.

It is quite common for couples to present themselves for screening – the patient and their anxious protagonist. After being screened themselves, it is not uncommon for the asymptomatic protagonist to benefit the most.

The inflexible nature of UK medical culture presents a problem. As medical scientists, we must answer a basic question about screening: 'what evidence of benefit is there?' Does it reduce mortality and / or morbidity? Despite the lack of definitive answers, my patient's desire for medical and cardiac screening never dampened. Most were aware that analyses of large group data might not apply to them, overlooking the benefit some individuals will get. Many saw screening as the dutiful thing to do, given their responsibility for others (their family and employees).

The wealthy mostly see the cost of screening as a small price to pay for a chance to preserve their life and to help maintain their chosen lifestyle. They will have made many similar 'common-sense', strategic judgements in business, based on much less evidence. They wanted to do anything they could to better the future for themselves, their families, and their employees. The 'public interest' and general good aspects of screening, were never their concern.

Screening patients are taking a gamble, when they put their money on the promise that early detection will lead to an improved prognosis. All my patients thought it a worthy gamble (given that they could easily afford it) and ignored the academic controversies doctors have about screening. In contrast to the need for evidence-based risk evaluation that is obligatory for medical scientists, my successful business patients, were those who would take a personal stand on issues of future significance without sufficient evidence. For them, decision making was an acknowledged art, awaiting scientific corroboration.

There are those who never give any thought to their car tyre pressures, engine oil level, or radiator fluid, before driving on a long road trip. Others give no thought to saving money for their retirement. Many believe that winning the National Lottery, or receiving a windfall from some distant relative, will provide the support they will need in later life. Instead, a little intelligent forethought might be better; at least this might be more reliable than hoping for the best, ill-informed gambling, disinterest, or absent-mindedness.

During the tragic bush fires in Australia in late 2019, Steve Harrison, a resident of Balmoral, New South Wales, con-

structed a ceramic coffin-sized kiln, just in case a bush fire overwhelmed his property. Because he put a fire extinguisher and several bottles of water in the kiln, many thought him over-anxious. His forethought saved his life. He hid inside the kiln for 30 minutes as a raging firestorm swept by.

Patient Demography

The socio-economic demographic of every medical practice will vary with postcode. Work location is important for doctors and nurses because there is a strong association between socio-economic grouping, disease prevalence, and clinical outcome. Both cancer and cardiac infarction incidence are three to five times more common in deprived areas. Poverty is a major aetiological factor in the occurrence and prognosis of all the major causes of death in the western world. It is thus a major medical and political issue that doctors and nurses must consider.

Two centuries ago, the rich were obese, and the poor were thin. The rich lived longer lives, and the poor shorter lives. To-day the rich are thin and the poor are obese, but the same difference in longevity remains. So, is longevity reduced most by being obesity or by living with poverty? The obvious scientific answer is poverty, but the current politically correct answer is obesity.

Being a Patient

Many patients are naturally apprehensive about medical interventions. Many see pharmaceutical drugs as harmful, with adverse effects on their immunity, gut bacteria, fertility and future health. Some who hold these views continue to drink alcohol, smoke and take street drugs, yet see no irony.

The acceptance of ideas can depend on need. Those desperate to find a cure may resign their objectivity and believe in myth and hearsay. The value we assign to scientific objectivity can vary with educational background. In my early years, I lived in a working class environment, and was only later let loose on the middle classes. I soon learned that hearsay, myth and the opinions of celebrities, were far less important to the educated and well-off.

Newly wealthy people seeking the excitement of something novel are especially prone to accept expensive, uncorroborated daft ideas; the need for self-indulgence acts as a strong bias. When trying to predict their future, they will readily follow in the footsteps of ancient rulers who visited Delphi. They wrongly thought the Oracle could predict their future. Many turn to spiritualists, astrology and Tarot card readers to predict their future, even if the advice they get is non-specific. In their quest for health and wealth, some will try healing crystals and the power of pyramids. All my oracle will tell me is that many myths, legends, conspiracies, and crazy theories sometimes contain a modicum of truth.

Nowadays, there are many websites which foster anti-medical, anti-science sentiment. Despite the advancements of science, superstition still gains acceptance. The effects of cold drafts, hot weather, barometric pressure, time of eating, vaccination and GM crops, all have their protagonists amongst those who dismiss scientific evidence.

Montenegro has a high proportion of smokers, yet what concerns Montenegrins most is the health risk of drafty conditions (Promaya).

*My patient, David L. had chronic back pain. He went
on holiday to Antigua, and for the first time in years,
became pain free. Since after returning to the UK his
quickly pain returned, he went back to Antigua for more
pain relief. In the end, repeated trips failed to help him.
He came to realise that it was partly the relief from
stress that had helped him initially, not the food or the
Caribbean waters in which he swam. I later discovered
the true cause of his back pain: ankylosing spondylitis.*

Big Pharma can contribute to patient distrust, while
trying to make bigger and bigger profits. For this reason they must promote their latest drugs, even when
the older and cheaper remedies are working well. The
apprehension some patients have about new drugs is
sometimes justified. Although doctors often try to
counter their concerns, patients expect their fears about
drugs to be acknowledged. While doing that, we should
also acknowledge the debt we owe to the pharmaceutical industry. They deserve our gratitude, since without
the many advances they have handed us, where would
modern medical management be?

Most patients bravely face our clinical conclusions and
medical advice, despite having to accept them on trust.
The closer they feel to disaster, the more willing they will
be to accept whatever we advise. I have always admired the
courage shown by many patients being approached by a
doctor holding a needle, endoscope, or scalpel. Coming to
deserve such trust depends a lot on how we engage with
patients and how we use the art of medicine. Accepting
that the reliable, reproducible results of scientific medicine
will work in the absence of a trusted doctor-patient rela-

tionship, patients still need confidence in those administering it. For this, the art of medicine is essential.

Two months after I started work as a surgical houseman (on the 30th July 1966), I admitted a 40-year-old man as an emergency. He experienced acute chest pain after swallowing a small dental plate with three false teeth attached. He had been watching the now famous FIFA World Cup football match in which England beat West Germany 4 : 2. At the final whistle, the patient jumped to his feet, and in his excitement, detached and swallowed his dental plate. It lodged half-way down his gullet.

Post-operatively, I told him we tried hard to remove his dental plate, but failed (using oesophagoscopy, under general anaesthetic). Regretfully, we had to proceed to a thoracotomy. 'That's alright', he said, 'It was worth it. England won!'

The vast majority of patients were once respectful of medical training, and the hours doctors and nurses worked. In 1966, junior doctors never counted these hours. Some of our consultants had served in the second world war, and would have not stopped work until they had dealt with every case. They expected us juniors to do the same. A recently expressed, bureaucratic point of view, challenged this. The question posed was, 'Who would want to be seen by a tired doctor?' My answer to that would be, 'I wouldn't mind if she was knowledgeable and dedicated to helping me.' During the COVID crisis, junior doctors again showed the same dedicated mettle. Meanwhile, bureaucrats with no need for dedication, retreated to the safety of their bunkers.

Patients give doctors and nurses their trust, with little more than faith to rely on. After all, we all have diplomas and certificates on our walls, stethoscopes draped around our necks, impressive tomes in our bookcases, and a lot of consulting room paraphernalia to inspire their confidence. Patients deserve capable, dedicated, energetic doctors and nurses who they can trust; their energy levels are important to their performance, but of secondary significance to their vocation and dedication when lives are at stake.

When the going gets tough, the tough get going. Those with devolved patient responsibilities who sit in offices from 9 to 5 for a six-figure salary, might think they understand our call to duty, our vocation and our dedication, but are they not deluded? Doctors and nurses, made of different stuff, deserve renewed respect; perhaps retraced back to what it was sixty-years ago.

Clarity and Confusion

Some patients get confused; some cannot understand, and some cannot remember what they were told. Although not demented, some may have a limited vocabulary and be barely literate. As big a problem is the inability we all have to concentrate after receiving bad news. Anxiety and fear diminish concentration. At such a time, the cultural differences between a doctor, nurse and a patient, might introduce further barriers to empathetic understanding. Unfortunately, not all doctors and nurses are versatile enough as 'performers' to adapt their language and approach to the needs of every patient.

If a patient feels that a doctor or nurse does not identify with them, or does not understand them, how will they feel able to accept them? Some will find reassurance in knowing that the GMC thinks them qualified to work. Ultimately, it is trust built on continuous exposure that best allows patients to agree with our suggestions of medical management.

Continuity is an invaluable commodity that continues to be relevant. Unfortunately, the NHS has steadily diminished its availability, but this is not yet so in private practice. In traditional private practices like mine, continuity is part of what patients paid for. It remains to be seen if this will continue to apply to private 'walk in' clinics. My concern is that if private medicine becomes incorporated like the NHS, profit and processing efficiency will become the focus, and the same lack of continuity will follow.

Continuity is not easily possible in A&E or in multi-handed GP practices. The trend for patients to attend one or the other, might demoralise those doctors and nurses who realise the crucial importance of continuity. Without enough time and continuity, practising the art of medicine becomes less feasible.

Managing Patient Information

How much detail should we reveal to each patient? I think it should depend on the patient and their circumstances. The amount divulged could be all, nothing, or an amount subject to judgement. In order to judge the amount that is appropriate, personal acquaintance with the patient is essential. Ideally, one will have formed an idea about the patient's knowledge, and their ability to understand, especially information that is technical. It is also essential to know their likely emotional reactivity, their anxiety, panic, bravery or stoicism in the face of upsetting information. One must know something of their ability to cope (with or without friends or family). These factors are all critical to how much information I would give to a patient, and how I would then manage them.

These days, there are doctors who insist on patients being told everything, regardless of the content and possible emotional impact. They will think there is no place for restricted disclosure, and no need to be concerned about the timing of information delivery. Their role is to divest themselves of responsibility and never to leave themselves open to criticism or accusations of non-compliance. These are the views of detached doctors, unhappy to take any responsibility for personal judgement, or to play a meaningful empathetic role.

The degree of clinical revelation suitable for each patient requires wise judgement. According to our regulators, total compliance with written guidelines and bureaucratic rules is now the *sine qua non* of clinical practice, not clinical judgement. This irreverent, ill-educated approach, neatly excludes the art of medicine and the judgements and management that flow from it. Total revelation of patient information is now the accepted norm, even though it wrongly presumes that all patients can understand it equally and are emotionally stable enough to cope with it. Clearly, this is nonsense, and clearly an extension of the political quest to convince us we are all equally able.

Information given as a matter of compliance, or as a legal requirement, can be inhumane. Duty stripped of humanity may be *de rigueur* when applying the rule of law, but it can be inappropriate for an attached doctor involved in improving the lives of sentient beings.

The act of divesting oneself of someone else's personal, possibly life-changing information, removes the need for personal responsibility. It can actually prove to be cathartic for the sheepish rule-followers among us, and those eager not to be caught using their own judgement by their peers and regulators. The dehumanised transfer of clinical information to a patient may well comply with 'best practice', but it can fall far short of what is in a patient's best interest.

By definition, every master of the art of medicine will know best how to exercise discretion; how much information to give, and how much to withhold, all of which he will vary from patient to patient. If the sovereignty and sacrosanct nature of medical practice in the lives of patients is any further eroded by corporatisation and bureaucracy, doctors can look forward to a bleak future - one in which they are trusted less and less to think for themselves and receive little or no respect for their clinical judgements.

As Confucius would have had it, it takes knowledge together with humanity (Ren:◻),for knowledge to qualify as wisdom.

The amount revealed to each patient, in how much detail, and at what time, are all important. Patients must always have enough information to assess the advice we give and be able to see sense in any course of action we advise. This process cannot be standardised. We must judge every action on its individual clinical merits. Adverse information can increase a patient's rate of demise; positive, encouraging information, can help speed their recovery. Information therefore has prognostic value. You would be right to ask for the evidence for this proposition, but posing the question might identify a clinically inexperienced, possibly detached observer.

'. . . it is diligence, and observation, and practice, and an
ambition to be the best in the Art   that must do it.'
                                          The Compleat Angler
Or the Contemplative Man's Recreation. Chapter 17. Izaak
                                                        Walton.

*My colleague, Dr. A. G, was trying to explain to an older
Jewish couple (Yiddish was their mother tongue), that he (the
patient, Mr. Cohen) needed a new pacemaker electrode. Dr.
A.G., told Mr. Cohen that the 'endocardial threshold of his
pacing electrode had been rising steadily'. Being told this,
and other jargon-based facts, left him and his wife looking
troubled.*

*My Jewish colleague, Dr. Paul K. from New York, was sit-
ting close by, listening with me to Dr. A. G's explanations.
We were all sitting in an open-plan, out-patient clinic, empty except for the five of us. Paul rose to his feet and wandered
over to Dr. A. G. and his patients. With a strong Bronx
(New York) accent he then said, 'Would 'ye mind if I said
a few 'woyids' to Mr. and Mrs. Cohen?' 'Be my guest', said
Dr. A.G, recognising the difficulty with communication he
was having.*

*Paul addressed the patient and his wife directly. Stand-
ing in front of them, with hands outstretched, he entreated
them, saying, 'Mr. and Mrs. Cohen, you're in good hands.
'Whad 'ye worried about?' The patient and his wife rose to
their feet, and with beaming smiles clasped Paul's hands,
and said, 'Thank-you doctor, that's all we wanted to know.'*

The types of patients a doctor will see are partly pre-selected; both practice location and its associated demography play their part. Other variables apply. If doctors and nurses work in private practice, business people will more often be their patients.

At least two types of business people present themselves as patients: company directors (or business owners), and their employees. Directors are usually the richer of the two, and are used to having their wishes granted. Their employees may have private medical insurance as a company perk. Directors will usually want to know all the facts and to be involved in the decision-making progress. Regardless of their position within the company, the facts you deliver will shape their further requests and expectations, and determine what they think of your management. Company employees will mostly be less critical and more accepting of all you say, and worried more about what medical revelation could mean for their job security.

Before the NHS existed, most hospital in-patients were there in receipt of charity. Medical and other staff expected them to be grateful and submissive. The NHS had only been running for 13-years when I entered medical school, and patients were still submissive, and doctors still rather formal and superior in their approach. On reflection, it has not been a bad thing for us to have loosened up, although it has made the jobs of some doctors more difficult. Instead of adopting a single, formal approach to patients, some doctors have had to master different approaches. Doctors must now earn the respect and faith of patients, whereas once it was automatic. Nurses have always enjoyed and deserved the unquestioned acceptance of patients.

Modern media has gained in divisive strength because it is unedited. This allows widespread comparisons to be made, opinions to be sought, and feedback to be circulated without reference to any authority. For doctors and nurses, there is now more to live up. There is also much more information to disquiet the apprehensive, once they wander beyond their level of understanding. It is good that media feedback and review can expose poor medical practice (albeit, with many false allegations), but it may not help those who are already apprehensive about their illness, or in fear of becoming ill.

The demography of the area in which doctors and nurses work will not only determine the likely prevalence of the diseases they see, but also the type of characters they will meet. Age, gender, education, socio-economic class, culture, race, family background, and wealth, all feed patient expectations, and the style of communication they will find acceptable. Being able to deal with these distinct groups requires sensitivity, and an art that needs practice. To succeed in UK medical practice now, versatility is essential.

Michael was a builder. His company built some of the major parts of the London Olympics stadia in 2012. He was a hard-working, worldly wise Irishman from Cork. He had no university degree, but was super-smart. One day he came 'to get his painful foot fixed'; he was suffering from acute gout. I explained about uric acid crystal formation in his joint tissues. I further explained about inflammation and the benefits of anti-inflammatory drugs, as well as about business stress as a causative factor. He said nothing much; thanked me and walked out.

I was later told by my receptionist what he said before leaving. 'I don't know what the f***ing hell he was talking about in there (my consulting room); something about crystals and inflammation. All I wanted was to get my foot fixed.'

I had wrongly assumed that Michael needed a pathophysiological explanation for his pain. I was later told that, where he came from in Ireland, most people still revere nurses and doctors and trust them without a second thought (not so often the case in the UK). His considerable trust in me, made my detailed explanations superfluous. For patients who trust their doctor this much, faith and trust can obviate the need for lengthy explanations.

The same level of trust in doctors still exists in many parts of the world. In the UK, after the cases of Dr. Harold Shipman and Lucy Letby, medical regulators came to regard trust in doctors and nurses as even more misplaced and dangerous than they did before. With the power vested in them, their mission is now to protect the public from the medical profession.

Clashes of Socio-economic Class

Differences in culture, education, and socioeconomic background will help define the mutual compatibility and acceptability of patient-doctor and nurse-patient relationships. The relationship will also depend on the mutual desire of each party to overcome any inter-personal barriers.

Although my upbringing was in what was then an under-privileged, working-class area of East London (Walthamstow), my family were self-employed and financially secure. My contemporaries at medical school were all middle-class, and except for two of us, ex-public school. In the course of our medical education, I noticed none of my fellow students struggling to communicate with the less privileged, but then unquestioned respect and deference existed towards medical students, doctors and nurses.

While at 'The London' (now the Royal London, in Whitechapel, London), we students were among the first to be taught 'communication' (1963) as a distinct subject. They taught us to engage with the Cockney patients who then outnumbered all other groups in Whitechapel, Bethnal Green, and Hackney (East London). The well-known affability and adaptability of Cockney's made communication easier. I have worked with both the under-privileged and the privileged, and have found no difficulty with either. It can be a challenge, however, to adjust to the mentality of those with long-standing family wealth and social privilege, although I only encountered it once.

In the 1970s, I was caring for a very wealthy business owner whose claim to fame was the invention of the first 'radiogram'. In the 1930s, his product was the first to combine a record-playing deck with a radio, enclosed in one smart piece of furniture. His father had been a furniture maker in Naples, and his sons both became manufacturers of their own well-known brand of furniture.

After having a stroke, he built a gymnasium in his house. He thought this would aid his recovery. When I next visited him, he had almost completely recovered. I thought it time for him to take a holiday. The question I put to him was innocent enough: 'Perhaps it's time for you to book a holiday?' To this, he jokingly pointed to his telephone, and said: 'I guess you know what that is Dr. Dighton? When I want to go on holiday, I lift the receiver and speak to my pilot. I might ask him to take me to my house in Bermuda or I might ask him

*to take me to my villa on Corfu. When you have your own
private jet, and several houses abroad Dr. Dighton, there is
no need to 'book' a holiday.'*

He taught me a lesson about the very wealthy I have
never again had to draw upon.

Sometimes, patients do not need to seek medical advice;
all they want is a certificate for work, or a chit for an eye
test. Conversation and discussion are not what they want;
their needs are administrative.

*Very early in my career, I did some GP locum work in
Stratford, East London (1967). The patients would come in
expecting to get a blue certificate, a yellow chit, a green form,
or a pink prescription. I cannot now remember now what
these various bits of paper were for. I tried to enquire about
their health, but was told not to bother. When asked by the
wise old Irish doctor (a Cork man), whose practice it was,
'How are you getting on young Dighton?' I replied, 'I have
found it rather difficult to talk to your patients'. Hearing
this, he leaned back, and with subdued exasperation, worthy
of any dramatic actor, took one long draw on his pipe. After
exhaling a diffuse cloud of tobacco smoke, he said something
I was never to forget: 'It's a grave mistake to talk to 'em!' He
had clearly gained the measure of his patients, and they of
him.*

What did he really mean? Was it just his Irish wit?
Perhaps he meant that having learned to converse with
educated people, he found it tiresome to deal with lesser
mortals. Maybe he had become weary of general practice,
having dealt too long with trivial matters. Was this why he
had minimised all of his communications with patients?
If doctors and nurses ever reach this point in their ca-

reer, they should retire or change jobs. Since an accurate diagnosis depends on obtaining a thorough history, any disinterest in communicating with patients will diminish a doctor's diagnostic ability and clinical effectiveness.

Victim or Patient?

As a lecturer in cardiology at Charing Cross Hospital in the 1970s, I worked with a charismatic doctor. Dr. P.N. was an inspired, insightful cardiologist, with ideas ahead of his time (and all of his colleagues). His interest was how changes in life circumstances, and in particular the stress of relationships, might cause cardiac infarction. He was certain that most heart attacks owed something to a mixture of anger, disappointment, and resentment (among many other responses). He observed that patients often denied personal responsibility for their fate; perhaps seeing it as disconnected, a weakness or an embarrassment.

When he first approached a patient in our coronary care unit, his first question was often: 'Who is trying to kill you?' A negative answer, a denial, a blank look, or a dismissive response, would cause him to say: 'Well, you'll just have to stay here until we find out. If we don't find out, how are you going to prevent another heart attack?'

Controversy over the connection between stress and disease continues today. How it affects the symptoms of established disease is less controversial, but not always considered by doctors (doctors are not social workers). Here are three anecdotes in historical order, suggesting that a connection exists between illness and stress.

- In late 1943, during the Second World War, Churchill was pushing his allies to continue the

Mediterranean offensive. The Allies voted against his plans. They mounted operation 'Overload', the campaign to invade northern France, before pushing on to Berlin. Churchill said he was being crushed between a Russian bear (Stalin), and an American elephant (Roosevelt). Churchill then developed pneumonia and had two small 'heart attacks'.

- In the film, 'A Nun's Story', a hypothetical relationship is suggested between stress and TB. It was based on the true life story of Marie Louise Habets, and came to cinemas in 1959 (Warner Bros.). The story depicts a nun (Sister Luke, played by Audrey Hepburn) conflicted by her religious duty and her calling to be a nurse. Having contracted pulmonary TB, her surgeon colleague (Dr. Fortunati, played by Peter Finch) suggests that her inner conflict is the disease, and TB merely a side-effect.

- During the fierce US presidential campaign of 2016 which she lost, Hillary Clinton's immune system may have reacted adversely. Like Churchill under stress, seventy-three years before, she developed pneumonia. Was her personal reaction to her failure responsible?

'Life' - The Play

'All the world's a stage, and all the men and women merely players: they have their exits and their entrances; and one man in his time plays many parts . . .'

Jacques, in *'As You Like It'*, Act 2, Scene 7

The roles played by doctors and nurses can affect the welfare of their patients.

With the same weight attached, weak elastic will stretch more than tough elastic and is more liable to snap. Using this simple physical analogy, the weight attached represents the physical *stress* and the amount of stretch the *strain*. As the stress increases and the strain reaches a critical point, the elastic will snap. This physical relationship, known to every GCSE physics student, has a bio-medical equivalent. Life events, like marriage, divorce, or bankruptcy (as stresses), can produce a spectrum of 'strain' effects, different for each individual. I have seen these events cause no change, or an increased susceptibility to infection, more migraine, resistant hypertension, worsening angina, psoriasis, worsening IBS, and depression. The bio-medical equivalent of elastic snapping is the sudden occurrence of a stroke or heart attack (the toughness of bio-medical elastic depends a lot on the patient's energy status. See later).

Stress can trigger some conditions, but perhaps only for those predisposed. Are these the responses of the weak? Do such responses never occur to those made of sterner stuff? Can genetic predisposition predict adverse responses to stress? Stress may not cause disease, but it can affect its progress.

Every patient will play many parts throughout their life, with their psychological state and illnesses influenced by their fellow 'players': those with whom they have relationships. Dr. P.N., at Charing Cross, specifically thought that responses to prevailing circumstances (psycho-pathophysiological and biochemical changes), could affect the course of coronary artery disease. He recognised that among the pertinent responses were a 'depleted' (or pro-inflammatory) immune system, exaggerated clotting, and changes in fluid dynamics (BP, and changes in blood viscosity associated with increased catecholamine output).

Dr. P.N. and I disagreed about the relative clinical contribution of stress to coronary atherosclerosis. He preferred to exclude mention of atherosclerosis from our presentations to other doctors, claiming he did not want his message diluted. The message he wanted to covey was that 'stress could worsen angina, and induce heart attacks'. He did not want to acknowledge the fact that without atherosclerosis, stress would not cause cardiac infarction. Cardiac infarction (a heart attack) is nearly always caused by fissuring of an atheromatous (cholesterol) plaque in a coronary artery. After this, platelet aggregation and clot formation (induced by stress in animals) can combine to block the artery. In the heart, this block can stop coronary blood flow and cause myocardial infarction (in the absence of an adequate bypass circulation). Stress undoubtedly reduces walking distance in those with angina. On that, we agreed.

For acutely ill patients, psycho-social-pathophysiological influences, culture, and character hardly need to be considered initially. In chronic conditions, they are more pertinent. Although enquiring into these factors can affect the consulting experience for both doctors and patients, it may not always change the outcome. Liken it to the ambience in a restaurant. It can alter the experience, but not change the taste of the food (although, according to chef Heston Blumenthal, it can. See neurogastronomy in 'Eater' 2016). Psycho-social enquiries can reveal important subsidiary factors that might in part explain a patient's demise. Although some doctors regard such enquiries as too personal, the information allows better targeted advice for individuals. In my experience, such enquiries strengthen the doctor-patient relationship.

In cases that do not respond to the usual management, doctors must consider asking: 'Is there any evidence of the patient's responses to previous stress?'

Can a patient's response to changing psycho-social factors alter the natural history of their condition? Difficult to manage cases, and those who do not improve, will often have relevant circumstance and relationship-related problems. Doctors should re-visit the clinical history, and broaden the enquiry (with permission) to include the views of friends, workmates, and relatives. At least they might recognise some contributing factors and understand why their improvement might be delayed. They might come to appreciate the medical value of social service agencies able to change a patient's circumstances for the better. There are, however, many patients with no intention of changing their circumstances, even if it offered them the prospect of improvement.

I will tell you how to cure your headaches and high blood pressure, Mr. Jones. It is obvious, but will be difficult for you. Divorce your wife. Tell all your demanding children to stand on their own two feet. Sell your business and retire

*to the Caribbean. At least go somewhere far enough away
from all those who aggravate and frustrate you. Make a
fresh start. You only have one life, Mr. Jones. Your life could
depend on you becoming 'a new man' with a normal blood
pressure.*

This form a conversation parodies one that Dr. P.N.
might have had at Charing Cross Hospital in the 1980s.
That few patients are likely to accept such advice doesn't
make it wrong; just difficult to follow. Patients will have
many reasons not to follow such advice. Some will have
emotional, inter-personal issues, and an unwillingness to
relinquish their responsibilities. Others will prefer to keep
their *status quo*, regardless of any threat to their life. Although the advice might seem a joke, it could stimulate
a patient to think about their situation and the reasons
for their continuing illness. By making such suggestions,
doctors can avoid responsibility for the patient's repeated
failure to improve. Expect some patients to react badly
to such advice and feel alienated. Others will respect the
attempt to help them.

An uncompromising approach can sometimes work
best when trying to achieve change. The aforesaid Mr.
Jones might acknowledge the points being made, but for
reasons related to trust, loyalty, commitment, responsibility and practicality, he may have no choice but to ignore
the advice. By so doing, he accepts his destiny, and will
continue to suffer. Giving such advice can bring respect for
a doctor who understands the patient's situation, and has
his best medical (if not social) interests at heart. This could
incur the resentment and anger of his friends and family.

Simple, off-the-cuff remarks can effect change; sometimes surprising change.

Ralph became a good friend of mine. He was a moderate smoker. His amiable, jovial character often lifted the spirit of those in his presence. His father had been a heavy smoker and died with bronchitis and emphysema. One day, Ralph developed bronchitis. After examining his chest, I made a casual remark. It was that his chest was 'going the same way as his father's' (note: I had decades of medical practice continuity with him, his father, and his grandchildren). I then thought no more of it.

Six months later, Ralph came to me for another examination. I asked a simple question: 'How many cigarettes do you smoke now, Ralph?' 'Smoke!' he replied indignantly, 'After what you said to me?' Somewhat perplexed, I enquired: 'What exactly did I say to you?' Ralph continued, 'The moment after you said that my chest was - going the same way as my father's, I stopped smoking forever! I would have been mad to continue.'

An unexpected life-changing response from one simple, off-the-cuff remark.

TATT (Tired All The Time), Fatigue and Exhaustion

Tiredness is perhaps the commonest of all symptoms.

Because all disease processes consume energy, tiredness will result if their advance. To understand physical tiredness, one must consider the amount of exercise undertaken (although, the toxic effects of disease can sometimes cause muscular tiredness and weakness). Mental tiredness is another matter, and less well understood. It can only come from spending more energy on brain functioning (solving problems, stress, anxiety, and obsessional behaviour) than on replenishing it. Replenishing happens with 'normal' sleep, although meditation and relaxation can also help. Sleep disorders (including those induced by stress) are common causes of tiredness. The more severe degrees of mental tiredness will influence the progress of every disease.

Anaemia, an under-active thyroid or diabetes are not the commonest causes of tiredness in the UK. The commonest causes relate to stressful circumstances, and associated sleep disturbances.

My former boss at Charing Cross, Dr. P.N., was an ex-army officer who had worked with the SAS and paratroopers. He had learned that fatigue affected a soldier's physical and mental performance, and that cognitive and emotional functioning can precede road traffic accidents. For this reason, lorry drivers have had their driving hours restricted. In the cardiac department of Charing Cross, we always assessed patient tiredness along with the contributing psycho-social factors.

Few doctors acknowledge tiredness as a relevant clinical factor, although all accept it as a secondary effect of illness. One year prior to cardiac infarction, many patients report increasing tiredness. This can be associated with an inability to sleep well while being preoccupied by stress. Since sleep-deprived rats have an increased liability to cardiac infarction, might this also apply to humans? Assuming it does, Dr. P.N's method for helping the exhausted was to replete their energy with sedated sleep (all night, and most of the day, for three consecutive days). If they had accompanying ECG changes (of ischaemia), he would diagnose 'pre-infarction syndrome' and anticoagulate them. Things have moved on considerably since then. These days, we would rather perform tests that reveal the coronary artery anatomy and take direct action to improve the blood flow.

While working at Charing Cross in the 1970s, I needed to define the degrees of tiredness our patients experienced.

- Simple tiredness, I defined as a feeling of depleted vitality (physical, or mental). There is a need for rest, but the potential still exists for them to perform well in response to everyday stimuli.

- Fatigue is tiredness without the potential for an increase in performance with motivation or stimulation.

- Exhaustion is tiredness, so extreme, that performance diminishes with stimulation. In this state, further stimulation risks physical and mental breakdown (an equivalent to elastic snapping when stretched too far). This failure can present clinically in various ways: panic attacks, psychotic episodes, cardiac infarction, uncontrolled hypertension (if predisposed), a minor stroke (TIA) or CVA (given predisposing factors). The most common outcomes, however, mostly involve an increased liability to infection (septicaemia, pneumonia, or the recurrence of herpes simplex, etc.). I have also seen patients with worsening psoriasis, and more frequent migraine accompanying stress induced tiredness.

In the Crimean War, Florence Nightingale noticed the fate of soldiers. If injured soon after arriving, their wounds

*quickly healed. Specifically, their wounds did not get infect-
ed and did not lead to fatal fever (septicaemia). She also
noted exhaustion amongst those who had fought for a long
time, and had suffered terrible climatic conditions in cold
muddy trenches. She noticed that they quickly succumbed to
septicaemia, even from one small scratch.*

Changes in immunity, hormone levels, and coagulation
can all occur with sleep deprivation, and can then affect
morbidity and mortality. Although mainly the subject
of anecdote, I have witnessed equivalent scenarios many
times. There is an important lesson to be learned here.
Tired, fatigued, or exhausted patients will not improve
without sufficient sleep. In the long-term, they will rarely
improve without some pertinent alteration in their circumstances, in particular those that led to their demise.
To be effective, any alterations made must prevent the recurrence of fatigue and exhaustion. During consultation,
it takes time to consider these energy factors; often more
time than doctors have available.

*Mrs. C. was an anxious person. Although she had had ab-
dominal pains for months, she complained of it only one
week before seeing me. My abdominal examination revealed a large, tender mass in her abdomen. She had a
partially obstructed bowel. Apart from an i.v. infusion, and
a Ryle's suction tube in her stomach, the surgeon I referred
her to left her untreated over the following weekend. He had
prior weekend arrangements.*

*The following week, he became strangely indecisive and in-
timated that performing the required operation was not for
him (the hospital staff and the family had harassed him
about his plan of action). Another surgeon operated on her
the next day, then six days after admission. At this stage,*

*the patient had suffered months of fear and worry, thinking
that she had cancer. Her days in the hospital had made
her even more worried. She was mentally and physically
exhausted. She died from septicaemia on the seventh post-op-
erative day. Histologically, the mass removed revealed a
combination of acute diverticulitis and colon cancer.*

Unnecessary delays amplified this patient's stress, anxiety, and fear. She was too long managed badly, and her
exhaustion completely ignored. Although not identifiable
at post mortem, any resulting reduction in her immune response would have significantly contributed to her death.

Alongside technical expertise, what competent doctor
would ignore individual human factors?

Nail in the Foot Syndrome

A nail in the foot will cause pain, eased only by its removal. Once removed, recovery can be quick.

*Josephine was in her 60s when I admitted her with high
blood pressure (consistently greater than 190/110). No medication reduced it. She told me she was the 'queen bee' of her
family-run furniture business. She also told me she was indispensable, and although she wanted to retire, she couldn't
let her family down.*

*After a bedside discussion that established these facts, I left
her to return to my consulting room. Coincidentally, her
husband then arrived. I requested a chat and suggested he
should let his wife retire, even though she was indispensable.
'Indispensable?', he said indignantly. 'I've been trying to get
her to retire for years. She simply refuses to go.' The solution
was now evident. 'Let's go back to her room', I said. 'Allow*

*me to say that I have persuaded you to let her go, while ac-
knowledging how difficult the situation will be for you.'
He agreed and allowed her to retire with her dignity in
place. Thereafter, it was easy to control her blood pressure
with much small doses of medication.*

What can seem to be a 'cure', or a substantial improvement in a medical condition, can sometimes result from modifying just one psycho-social factor.

Conditions with a stress related, psychoneurotic element, commonly present with tiredness (TATT: **T**ired
All **T**he **T**ime), and/or depression. As a doctor trained
in hospital medicine and cardiology, I did not readily
take to psycho-social evaluation. I became convinced
of its value once I had witnessed the consequences of
ignoring it. Sometimes, one cannot treat patients appropriately without knowing what is most important
to them in their lives.

Impasse

- ***Doctor:*** *'I am very pleased to tell you, Mrs.
  Smith, that all your tests have been returned
  within normal limits. Therefore, there is nothing wrong with you'* (despite all your symptoms).

- ***Patient:*** *'Why then do I feel so ill, tired, and
  weak, doctor?'* (meaning you have failed to convince me you know what you are talking about).

This doctor now has options:

1: On the presumption that he has missed something, he can return to square-one, retake the history, and re-examine the patient.

2: He can dismiss the patient with the implication that she is wasting his valuable time.

3: He could survey her psycho-social landscape for aetiological clues.

4: He could refer her to an appropriate colleague. Beware, though, if that colleague is not interested in circumstances as aetiological agents, she might return feeling no better. If she returns, she may want to discuss all that your colleague said. I have always found this unacceptable. I preferred to refer my patients to colleagues who would leave no loose ends for me to resolve and explain.

The Games People Play

Should one seek solitude or a relationship? Although a common lifestyle choice, attraction may draw us in, but few then give much thought to the consequences. Many engage in a relationship hoping it to be loving, fulfilling and long-term. Sadly, that is not always the case; relationships all too frequently result in lifelong conflict. Many still prefer this to isolation and loneliness.

Relationship problems are among the commonest causes of stress, potentially changing the natural history of a disease and its management. Knowing about a patient's relationships can, therefore, be of clinical relevance. They sometimes explain recalcitrance, non-compliance and therapeutic failure.

In 1964, psychiatrist Eric Berne wrote his landmark book (*The Games People Play*), describing the interplay between people. It is a *must* read for anyone interested in understanding why people behave as they do.

Emma Morano, from Lake Maggiore, Italy, was born on the 29th of November 1899. As the oldest living person on Earth in 2017 (then 117-years-old), she gave credit to being single, going to bed early, and eating three eggs every day (one cooked, two raw). She thought her wisest move was to leave her violent husband in 1938.

As a pastoral exercise, someone once asked me to evaluate the compatibility of a couple intending to marry. Apart from mutual physical attraction, the long-term stability of relationships depends on each participant getting their cognitive and emotional needs fulfilled by their partner. Why else would anyone want another person to share their life? So, can we measure compatibility reliably?

Mr. J. owned an international engineering company. His headstrong 20-year-old son had insisted on marrying a young woman he met on holiday. The advice of both his parents was for them to wait a while, and get better acquainted. The marriage lasted three months and cost the family over one million pounds.

When his son came home with another young woman he intended to marry, his father became perturbed. Given the potential cost of another failed marriage, Mr. J. insisted on some evidence for their compatibility, and much more information about his girlfriend and her family. He engaged a private detective for the purpose. He worried about losing his son and even more money.

He asked me for help. After some research, I found a rather old compatibility questionnaire: the FIRO B test (Funda-

mental Interpersonal Relations Orientation; 'B' for Behaviour). William Schutz introduced it in 1958. The couple agreed to take the test, but I insisted they came to see me separately on the same day. I didn't want them to confer. The results surprised both me and Mr. J. They strongly supported the view that the couple were a perfect match. When last I asked, they were still happily married after 25-years. Mr. and Mrs. J. now have three grandchildren.

Schultz designed the FIRO B test to assess the inter-relationships of US air force flight crew. While flying, near disasters had occurred when inter-personal conflicts on the flight deck diverted the crew's attention. The test provided them with a useful, semi-quantitative measure of relationship compatibility. As a result, the US air force chose more compatible flight crews.

There is a presumption in scientific circles that the age of any research done somehow affects its veracity, reliability, usefulness and relevance. These assumptions all need to be reviewed.

The FIRO-B test is still available. It assumes that we all have three 'core' needs to be satisfied, or otherwise rejected within a relationship. These needs are for *affection, control, and inclusion*. If one partner wants to give affection, compatibility requires that their partner wants affection (albeit subconsciously). Likewise, a controlling person is best matched with one whose desire is to be controlled. Inclusion refers to shared interests, outlook and cultural values. Inclusion is the weakest of the three compatibility factors. Relationships can survive mismatches of inclusion. Affection and control are strong factors binding people together. Any mismatch in either will quickly lead to estrangement.

The test is old, but has lost none of its predictive power. Too few of us understand why we feel compatible, incompatible, happy, or unhappy in the company of some others, including doctors and nurses. Too few know about Schultz's valuable work, and do not appreciate the true nature of the 'chemistry' they feel (or do not feel) with others.

A note about current compliance. No cardiologist in the UK could now officially employ such a questionnaire. A doctor not holding a certificate for clinical psychology, or relationship counselling, would not be acceptable. Regulators would question a doctor's qualification to use such a psychological instrument, and would regard those who do as a maverick needing to be replaced or watched closely.

Specialisation and certification have brought about the de-skilling of doctors. Doctors must now stick rigidly to their certification. That means fewer doctors can claim to be generalists, able to deal with all-comers. That has depleted the knowledge and experience base of medical practitioners. One consequence is that patients now find it harder to find a doctor who can help them.

Thinking for oneself and using one's initiative is key to succeeding with challenging clinical cases, and practising personalised medicine. It is not possible to standardise individualisation. For intelligent, experienced professionals, doing what has to be done for individual patients supersedes blindly following rules, regulations, and generalised guidelines. Blocking initiative and free thinking with too many rules and regulations diminishes the practice of medicine in the eyes of patients, but improves it in the eyes of bureaucrats. Why did doctors not resist the introduction of corporate standardisation techniques that belong in baked-bean factories?

When Matt Hancock was Minister of State for Health, he commended those doctors who performed inventively during the COVID-19 pandemic. Doctors and nurses functioning without bureaucratic control must have surprised him. (BBC 4, The Andrew Marr Show, 5/7/20).

What must we do to educate medical bureaucrats and health ministers so they fully appreciate the work and import of doctors and nurses? Perhaps they should all have medical degrees and be competent practitioners. My advice is to replace them all as soon as possible before the NHS becomes completely unfit for purpose. Although it is failing fast, it still pays legions of executives, among them a large number of lawyers and those with MBAs, taking home large six-figure salaries.

Patients in the UK who want to survive medical practice are going to have to re-think the value they assign to the NHS as it is managed currently, and revalue doctors and nurses whose work is dedicated to improving and saving their lives.

BIBLIOGRAPHY

Aeschylus (*The Persians*, 441 BC)

'Allo.'Allo! (BBC TV Series; 1982 – 1992). Writers: David Croft, Jeremy Lloyd and Paul Adam.

Armfield, Harry. *Cool. The Complete Handbook* (19 86).Pavilion Books.

Asher, Dr. Richard (1972) . *Talking Sense*. Pitman Books.

Augustine, Saint. *Confessions*.

Berne, Eric. (1964). *The Games People Play*. Grove Press.

Bible, The(The King James' Bible).

Chester v Afshar: [2004] UKHL. 41.

Company of Parish Clerks in London: *'Twenty died of parental 'Grieffe'.*

Crisp-Crown Index. Middlesex Hospital Questionnaire, Crisp, A.H., Crown, S. B.J.Psychiatry (1966); 112: 917-23

Culpeper, Thomas. (1515 – 1541) *'no man deserved to starve to pay a proud, insulting, domineering physician'.*

Dawkins, Richard (2019). *Outgrowing God. OUP*

Dekker, Thomas (1603). *Sweet ContentThe Pleasant Comoedy of Patient Grissill.*

Dighton, D.H. (2005) *Eat to Your Heart's Content.* HeartShield.

Dighton, D.H. (2007) *HeartSense.* HeartShield.

Dighton, D.H. (2023). *The NHS. Our Sick Sacred Cow.* Medicause.

Doctor in Clover, (Film. Rank Organisation, 1966).

'Eater' (Feb 19, 2016) Chef Heston Blumenthal. It's all about flavor perception. Whitney Filloon.

Eliot, George. *Middlemarch (1871).*

Eliot, T. S. (1926). *The Hollow Men* .

Enfield, Harry (1990). *The Slobs.* BB2.

Fish Called Wanda, A (Film, MGM. 1988).

Flick, Otto Herr, played by Richard Gibson. TV series *'Allo. 'Allo!*

Forsyth, Mark. (2013). *The Elements of Eloquence.* Icon Books.

Friedman, M.; Rosenman, R. (1959). *Association of specific overt behaviour pattern with blood and cardiovascular findings.* Journal of the American Medical Association. 169 (12): 1286–1296.

GMC. (2024). *Good Medical Practice.*

Granger, Dr. Kate. *'#HelloMyNameIs'*

Hardy, G. H. (1940) *A Mathematician's Apology.*

Harari, Yuval. *Homo Deus.* (2015). Random House.

Harvey, Dr. William.(1628). *Exercitatio Anatomica de Motu Cordis et Sanguinis in Animalibus.*

Hibbert, Christopher (2001). *Queen Victoria: A Personal History.* Harper Collins.

Hobbes, Thomas. (1651) *The Leviathan'.*

Illich, Ivan. (1999) *The Obsessional with Perfect Health.*

Illich, Ivan (1974) *Limits to Medicine: Medical Nemesis.* Re: *'narcissistic scientism'.*

I'm All Right Jack'.(1959).(Charter Film Productions, Boulting Brothers).

Jenkins, Simon. The Guardian 25/8/2017: *'It is more important to make what is important measurable, than to make what is measurable important.'*

Johnson. Dr. Julian P. (1939). *'The Path of the Masters'* (The Science of Surat Shabd Yoga), written by a (Radha Soami Satsung Beas / Punjab).

Langely, J.N. Brain; Part 1. (1903). *The Autonomic Nervous System.*

Life of Brian, The (1979), HandMade Films, and Python (Monty) Pictures.

Machiavelli, Nicoló. (1532) *The Prince.*

Marsh, Carl. (1939). *The Path of the Masters.* Radha Soami Satsung Beas (Punjab, India).

McChrystal, General Stanley A. (2015) *Team of Teams. Tantum Books.*

M*A*S*H; TV series; 20th Century Fox television.

Maraolo et al. (2017). *Doctors working long hours. Personal life and working conditions of trainees and young specialists in clinical microbiology and infectious diseases in Europe: a questionnaire survey.*Eur. J. Clin. Microbiol. Infect. Dis. doi:10.1007/s10096-017-2937-4).

Middlesex Hospital Questionnaire (MHQ), Crisp, A. H., Crown, S. B.J.Psychiatry (1966); 112: 917-23).

Minghella, Dominic. *Doc Martin*. Played by Martin Clunes in the UK, TV series (2004-2009).

NICE. National Institute for Health and Care Excellence: NICE Guidelines.

Nightingale, Florence. Fee, E., Garofalo, M.E. *Florence Nightingale and the Crimean War*. Am. J. Public Health (2010); 1591.

Ovid: *Metamorphoses*; Book III:402-436).

Palin, Michael. (BBC 1997). *Full Circle, trip of the world*.

Pauling, Linus. (1901 – 1944).The Linus Pauling Institute. Oregan State University.

Pope, Alexander (1711). *An Essay on Criticism*. Part 2. Anodos Books (2017).

Rushdie, Salman (1988). *The Satanic Verses*. Viking Penguin.

Sacks, Dr. Jonathon (2018). Former UK Chief Rabbi, *The Power of Praise*.

St. Paul. New Testament Epistles. Corinthians.

The Summa Theologiæ of St. Thomas Aquinas (1225-1274).

School for Scoundrels. (Film. Associated British Picture Corp., 1960).

Schiller, Friedrich. *The Maid of Orleans [Die Jungfrau von Orleans]*, Act III, sc. vi (1801) [tr. Swanwick]*Mit der Dummheit kämpfen Götter selbst vergebens*

'Against ignorance the Gods strive in vain.' (1801).

Schutz, W.C. (1958). FIRO: *A Three Dimensional Theory of Interpersonal Behaviour*. New York, NY: Holt, Rinehart, & Winston.

Semmelweis, Dr. Ignaz Philipp . *Hungarian gynaecologist who discovered that when doctors washed their hands after dissection, it prevented puerperal fever.*

Shakespeare, William: *As You Like It (Act 1, Scene 1).*

Shakespeare, William. *As You Like It*, Act 2, Scene 7. 'All the world's a stage'.

Shakespeare, William. *Hamlet: Act 3, Scene 1.* '*The insolence of office . . .*'

Shrek. (Film. Universal Pictures, 2001).

Shulchan Aruch, The. (1563)Joseph Karo.

Tversky, A., Kahneman, D. (1973). *Judgement under Uncertainty: Heuristics and Biases.* Hebrew University. Jerusalem.

Theophrastus. *The Characters of Theophrastus*. Book.

Walton, Izaak. (1653): *The Compleat Angler.* 'Those restless thoughts which corrode the sweets of life.'

Waugh, Evelyn. *Decline and Fall.* (1928). 'We school-masters must temper discretion with deceit.' *Words of* Dr. Fagan to Mr. Pennyfeather.

Wiseman, Richard. Psychologist. *The MegaLab Truth Test*, Nature, 373, 391. 'One third of us lie every day.'

Xenophon's Dialogue, *Ieron (Hiero), written in the 4th century BC* (Chapter 7, section 3),

INDEX